# BLIND
## *to the*
# MIND

*Illness Beyond Disease*

SUDHIR KOTHARI, NEUROLOGIST
KINJAL GOYAL, PSYCHOLOGIST

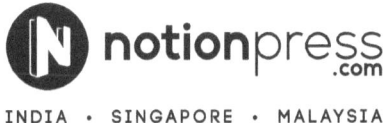

INDIA · SINGAPORE · MALAYSIA

## Notion Press

No.8, 3rd Cross Street,
CIT Colony, Mylapore,
Chennai, Tamil Nadu – 600004

First Published by Notion Press 2021
Copyright © Sudhir Kothari, Kinjal Goyal 2021
All Rights Reserved.

ISBN
Hardcase 978-1-63745-417-6
Paperback 978-1-63806-675-0

This book has been published with all efforts taken to make the material error-free after the consent of the author. However, the author and the publisher do not assume and hereby disclaim any liability to any party for any loss, damage, or disruption caused by errors or omissions, whether such errors or omissions result from negligence, accident, or any other cause.

While every effort has been made to avoid any mistake or omission, this publication is being sold on the condition and understanding that neither the author nor the publishers or printers would be liable in any manner to any person by reason of any mistake or omission in this publication or for any action taken or omitted to be taken or advice rendered or accepted on the basis of this work. For any defect in printing or binding the publishers will be liable only to replace the defective copy by another copy of this work then available.

Yesterday I was clever, so I wanted to change the world.

Today I am wise, so I am changing myself.

— Rumi

# Contributors

- **Dr Manish Agarwal**
  M.S.(ortho); D.N.B(ortho), Diploma in tissue banking (NUH, Singapore)
  Orthopaedic Oncosurgeon

- **Dr Prasad Ramkrishna Chandragiri**
  Medical Education, Advertising, and Medical writing

- **Prof Dr Milind V Kirtane**
  MBBS, M.S., D.O.R.L, DSc(Hon)
  Otorhinolaryngologist & Neurotologist

- **Manisha Lobo**
  M.Sc. (Biotechnology)
  Medical Education and Medical Communications

- **Dr Yash Lokhandwala**
  MBBS, MD, DM
  Cardiologist

- **Dr Sanjeev Mehta**
  MD, FCCP, FAPSR
  Pulmonologist, Specialist in Chest, Allergy, and Sleep medicine

- **Dr Sandeep Patwardhan**
  M.S., D.Orth
  Paediatric Orthopaedic Specialist

- **Dr Uday Phadke**
  MD, DNB, DM, FACE
  Consultant in Endocrinology and Diabetes

- **Dr Anantbhushan Ranade**
  MBBS, MD (Medicine)
  Medical Oncologist

- **Dr Vinay Thorat,**
  MD, DNB, DM, PhD
  Gastroenterologist

- **Dr Aniruddha Vyas**
  MBBS, MD, DM
  Cardiologist

- **Dr Jaini Lodha Bhandari**
  MBBS, M.S.(ENT), DNB
  Otorhinolaryngologist

# Contents

| | |
|---|---|
| *Foreword* | 9 |
| *Acknowledgements* | 15 |
| *Introduction* | 19 |
| **Chapter 1** An Introduction to Psychosomatics: Mind Your Body | 21 |
| **Chapter 2** Pain: A Mind Game | 52 |
| **Chapter 3** Headache: The Aching Mind | 65 |
| **Chapter 4** Gastroenterology: The Gut Feeling | 81 |
| **Chapter 5** Endocrinology: Don't Shoot the Messenger | 94 |
| **Chapter 6** Cardiology: Straight from the Heart | 110 |
| **Chapter 7** Dizziness: A New Spin | 123 |
| **Chapter 8** Tinnitus: Ring out the Old | 143 |
| **Chapter 9** Pulmonology: Breathe in, Breathe out | 148 |

| | | |
|---|---|---|
| **Chapter 10** | Orthopaedics: A Bone to Pick | 166 |
| **Chapter 11** | Oncology: A Matter of Growth | 185 |

*Conclusion*     *201*

# Foreword

**Prof Jon Stone MBChB FRCP PhD**

Honorary Professor of Neurology,
Centre for Clinical Brain Sciences,
University of Edinburgh,

Edinburgh, UK

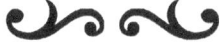

As a junior doctor beginning my training in UK Neurology in the early 1990s, I began to encounter patients that were not in my neurology textbooks. They didn't appear in lectures, research or training, except perhaps as a final option in a grand round when all else had been considered. They had the same symptoms and disability as my other patients with multiple sclerosis, epilepsy and stroke, but no abnormalities on their tests - their problems were 'non-organic', although now I would use the term Functional Neurological Disorder (FND). And there were so many of them!

What baffled me most was the attitude of many of the doctors towards them. Senior consultants whose acumen and professionalism I was keen to emulate appeared to struggle to know what to say or do with them. Their approaches to the problem in front of the patient were strikingly varied although often unconvincing: 'I think you must have some microscopic inflammation that the scans are not showing', 'It's not a neurological problem so I can't help', 'Have you been stressed recently – that might be causing your weak leg?'. Mostly they discharged the patient as soon as possible. Even some of the psychiatrists had little interest. Behind closed doors neurologists would talk about patients needing 'face saving' treatment, something I've always considered an implicit suggestion of wilful exaggeration, or would be more explicit about the problem being 'bogus'. Some more senior neurologists who tended to attract more such patients as 'difficult cases' clearly had more sophisticated views and often a desire to help but approaches often seemed to be ad hoc and passed down, not systematised or researched. Patients were frequently left baffled or upset and rarely seemed to get treatment.

I was baffled too, as I read more about functional disorders and their long and tortuous history in medicine, I couldn't understand how we had got here. Why were my supervisors so expert in most of their role but so often inept in relation to such a common part of their job. Worse still, why weren't they more curious about these people's suffering? Neurologists in the late 19th century and early 20th century like William Gowers, Henry Head and Jean-Martin Charcot had taken a keen interest in hysteria, as these disorders were known then. Their scientific and clinical observations stand the test of time very well, but something weird had happened after the first world war.

Medical progress is meant to be linear with knowledge accumulating, each generation standing on the shoulder of the one before. But instead, knowledge about functional disorders seemed to have gradually disappeared over time, fading from the neurology curriculum to such an extent that historians like Edward Shorter thought the disorders had also disappeared.

I am fortunate to be part of a renaissance of interest in this field over the last 20 years that I share with many colleagues. Functional disorders are fascinating. They challenge us to think about the brain, mind and body in new ways and relinquish assumptions that are embedded in much of our language and culture. Their history mirrors change in philosophy and science over thousands of years. As a subject to study, I am glad that I will never truly complete my understanding of functional disorders. To understand the nature of all the varied ways in which a human being's nervous system and body can malfunction, requires a complete understanding of what it is to be human in the first place.

We are at an exciting time for the science of these disorders – that is clear. Our models of brain and body function especially those around the brain as a predictive organ, an organ of allostasis and interoception, which is doing its best to anticipate and adapt to the world around it, are providing exciting new ways of thinking about how brain/body dysfunction might arise. Working in FND, I'm able to promote a new 'rule in' approach to diagnosis based on physical signs such as Hoover's sign.

Functional disorders are arguably an expected consequence of these models of brain function, and our new transparent approach to diagnosis and treatment correctly sits neither wholly in neurology or psychiatry. International collaborative research in functional disorders, encouraged by societies such as the FND society or the Rome foundation, is now much more common, and there is increasing evidence base treatment.

At the same time, we are beginning to see a slow turnaround in the neglected areas within medical practice that were so obvious to me as a trainee. One of my early mentors was worried that I could be wasting a promising career with my interest in functional disorders and psychiatry. Now it's a topic that is finding its way back into the mainstream, although we still have a very long way to go. Many patients with disorders at the interface between internal medicine and psychiatry still routinely experience poor standards of diagnosis and treatment, or harm from misdiagnosis. Our language and thinking also remain problematic. As I've described, some of my neurological trainers were, like the title of this book, 'blind to the mind', but if, as I think neuroscience shows us, that dualism is wrong – and the mind and brain are one – should we even use the words mind and brain?

We all struggle with these issues in writing about this topic.

It is in this context that I welcome this practical and multidisciplinary volume from Sudhir Kothari and Kinjal Goyal along with colleagues from many specialities. The text is written in the true original spirit of psychosomatic medicine. The word psychosomatic is much misunderstood and maligned, both by health professionals and patients. Its original meaning was as a bidirectional word that intended to convey not only the influence of cognitions and emotions on the body, but the opposite too – how the body influences the mind and brain. Their text cover not only the topic of functional disorders across an impressive range of symptoms and specialties but also the way in which conditions like cancer or heart disease are moderated by cognition and emotion.

They have produced a highly readable text, with vivid case descriptions that take you right in to the consulting room. It's especially apt that Drs Kothari and Goyal, a neurologist, and psychologist, have come together to provide a unified approach to these disorders, showing how we need to blur the dualist boundaries of our job titles and training if we want to help our patients with disorders that don't fit neatly into our conventional medical categories. It's also important to see these disorders discussed in the context of Indian rather than European or US practice. Although the main themes are universal, there are specifics, such as the spectre of femicide, or the hidden use of 'ganja' by an Indian priest that are clearly very different. I'm not convinced that the phenomenology of physical symptoms changes much around the world or across time, but the way people respond to them, and the challenges they face in making sense of them are undoubtedly shaped strongly by the culture they occur in.

In my own development as a neurologist, I found myself modifying the rigid history taking style I was taught in the 1980s to better suit the patients I was seeing with FND. I started asking my patients what ideas they had about what was wrong, and their experiences with other health professionals, especially when it had gone wrong. I learned to be aware of the potential influence of depression, anxiety, adversity and personality, but also hopefully not to rush to invade an individual's privacy or be tempted to 'solve them like a puzzle'. Eventually it dawned on me that this approach had rubbed off on my general neurology work. Neurology and medicine generally were more interesting and rewarding for it.

We desperately need leaders within each speciality of medicine, and health professionals in general, to help others wake up to the limitations of a purely molecular or structural approach to human health. I hope one day we may look back with some embarrassment at how we treated our patients who happened to have functional disorders that we couldn't yet diagnose using technology, but which were clinically staring us in the face the whole time if we only chose to listen. It's wonderful that Dr Kothari, Dr Goyal and colleagues are setting that example with this book, and also providing so many practical ideas to help broaden their readers' attitude and clinical approach.

*You can read more about Dr Stone's work at: https://neurosymptoms.org*

# Acknowledgements

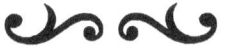

As Albert Schweitzer once said, "At times, our own light goes out and is rekindled by a spark from another person." It is to all those people who rekindled our spark, that we are truly grateful.

This book was a project undertaken by us nearly three years ago. We were inspired by various people: doctors who blazed a trail in psychosomatic approaches in their practice and others who turned a blind eye to it, patients who willingly accepted the role of their mind in their disease-illness spectrum and those who shrugged it off. Our own practice, as a neurologist and psychologist, gave us the privilege to build upon our experiences and learning, and in amalgamating those into a book.

At the outset, we would like to extend our warmest gratitude to our esteemed contributors. Not only did they take the time out of their busy practices to contribute to this book, but they also allowed us to brainstorm with them even before the book had any real structure. Their inputs in the respective chapters have added a whole new dimension to our understanding and explanation of psychosomatic ailments. We have learnt an incredible amount from all these stalwarts and will always cherish the process we have shared with them.

We would also like to thank Dr Jagdish Hiremath, a dear friend and colleague who took time out to read through some chapters and offer objective and constructive ideas on making them better. We extend our gratitude towards Deeksha Kalyani, Dr Ashutosh Chauhan, Dr Chetan Pradhan, Katya Hegde and Dr Anjali Bhimrajka for reading through and giving their unbiased inputs on various chapters as they were being written. A warm note of appreciation to Dr Jon Stone and Dr Diego Kaski for sparing their valuable time for discussing certain concepts in the book and offering their inputs. Having a Foreword by Dr Stone has indeed been an absolute honour. We are also grateful to Meghana Dharap, who read through our initial drafts and gave her valuable editorial suggestions. Our deepest gratitude towards Sanyukta Kothari for conceptualizing the cover design and helping us to transform our ideas into an image.

We would also like to thank all the patients who gave us their consent to use their case studies in the book. Although the details of the cases have been used with their informed consent, their names have been changed to protect their privacy.

Our families, especially our better halves, Rajesh Goyal and Anjali Kothari, deserve our warmest thanks for being unconditionally supportive as we stared at our screens for hours on end, trying to will the sentences into the right order!

We would like to extend our appreciation to the team at Notion Press for their help and patience with this book. As the pandemic struck, we were all caught unawares and our submission deadlines faltered. But all through, the publishing team stood by our side, accommodating every delay and making the process as smooth as possible.

As co-authors, we are thankful for having the opportunity to learn from each other and to be able to use this knowledge for better helping our patients in the future.

# Introduction

By Dr Sudhir Kothari

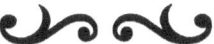

This is a book bringing out in the open, something we all know and yet don't know; the role of the mind in disease and illness, about medically unexplained symptoms; where the problem lies with the mind, but the body cries out. Distress and suffering are genuine, and yet, often all that the patient gets is "It's all in your head" or "Don't worry; there is nothing wrong. Just try to relax." No wonder there is dissatisfaction, and a lingering doubt as to whether another doctor or further testing is the answer. We are making an attempt to sensitize doctors and patients to psychosomatic illness, in various fields of medicine.

No one likes unexplained symptoms, neither the patient nor the doctor. The problem exists, in a large part, because we are shy or hesitant to think of the mind in a person with symptoms related to the body, like pain or fatigue. We somehow forget how much the mind can affect our body.

One cannot ever tease the mind out from the body; you always treat the person.

For me, managing *migraine* was where the rubber met the road. Migraine became the cusp between Neurology and Psychology, between the brain and the mind. Reading the book 'Migraine' by Oliver Sacks gave me a totally new perspective and I stopped looking at migraine as a disease. I looked at each patient as an individual; delving into his/her personal life. I realized that helping the person be happier, satisfied and relaxed would help the migraine. I learned the nuanced difference between disease, illness and sickness, one headache at a time.

Once I saw how rewarding the approach was in migraine, I started to look at and gradually learned to respect the mind in all of medicine. Psychosomatic disorders no longer became a stepchild, where I was stingy with empathy and validation. A doctor is made to be a healer and to address all human suffering, not just disease.

I am very happy that Dr Kinjal thought of us writing this book, as I have thoroughly enjoyed becoming a student of the mind in neurology and all these medical disorders.

I have learned now that disease is what I see as a doctor, illness is what the patient suffers while sickness is what the family or society considers it to be. I feel that as doctors and as a society, we all need to be more mindful of functional disorders and treat such sufferers with empathy. It is time, we completely reject dualistic thinking and treat the mind and body as one.

# CHAPTER 1
# An Introduction to Psychosomatics: Mind Your Body

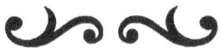

### A brief history

There is a large area of misunderstanding about what comprises psychosomatic ailments. Many equate them with malingering or factitious disorders; the so-called 'fake' symptoms, which are, to some degree at least, manipulated by patients. As awareness about such disorders grew, a new term came into being: 'Medically Unexplained Physical Symptoms' or MUPS. Every doctor almost invariably came across physical symptoms that no tests or imaging could account for. Kurt Kroenke and others showed that MUPS often showed an overlap with anxiety, depression, and somatization.

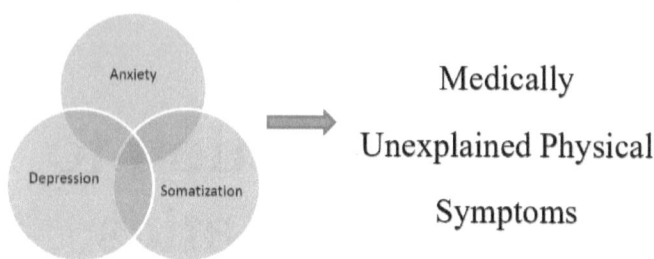

It was realized that it was not uncommon for anxiety and depression to present with physical symptoms rather than mental symptoms.

The concept of MUPS made it easier for doctors to factor in emotional issues like anxiety and depression into the diagnosis of an ailment that had physical symptoms at the fore. Over the years, however, physicians realized that although the concept of MUPS provided a vague idea of the overlap between the patient's mind and body, it provided no answers or solutions to the problem at hand. The label of a symptom or a symptom complex being medically unexplained didn't really help with the treatment beyond a point.

The Diagnostic and Statistical Manual, or the DSM V, changed some of the nomenclature as well as diagnostic criteria of psychosomatic ailments to bring more clarity and to provide a clearer direction for treatment. It has classified them into the four categories, Somatic symptom disorders, Illness anxiety disorders, Functional Neurological Disorders and Factitious disorders.

DSM V no longer makes it mandatory to seek for and demonstrate evidence of stress or psychological disorder. In any case, when looked for, it is rare that one does not find it.

## Which diseases are psychosomatic?

To a large extent, most diseases involve both, the mind and body. Some affect the body more, some the mind more, and some affect both more or less equally.

There is a mental aspect to every physical disease. How a person views his or her disease is variable. Pain threshold also varies from person to person. Other psycho-social factors also play an important role in the perception of diseases. For example, a person may hobble to work despite a fracture in the foot, while another may be unable to even walk within the house with a muscle cramp. The same is true for migraines. Although it is hard to objectively judge the scale of pain an individual is experiencing, some people tend to be able to bear a migraine with just an analgesic, while some are unable to carry out even the most basic activities despite medication.

There can also be physical effects from mental illnesses. For example, a person who is severely clinically depressed may not eat well or may have problems sleeping. Sometimes, personal hygiene takes a backseat too. All of this can lead to physical problems.

However, the term psychosomatic disorder is mainly used to mean *a physical disease that is thought to be caused, or made worse, by mental factors*. Mental factors can cause physical symptoms in the absence of any physical disease (for example, stress leading to non-cardiac chest pain or anxiety leading to breathlessness when the lung function is normal). Having a physical disease does not preclude another superimposed psychosomatic disorders. Similarly, mental factors can worsen the symptoms of an existing physical ailment (for example, periods of intense stress can cause a spike in blood pressure, worsen existing cardiac arrhythmias, cause flare-ups in stomach ulcers, etc. despite the patient being on medication that has proven its efficacy in the past).

If we knew enough about the mind, body, and medicine, we would be able to clearly distinguish symptoms and always place them on the correct side of the border, if in fact, there was one. It is, in fact, not easy to mark the borders between the mind and body at all. Most diseases have strong overlaps between the mind and the body and cannot be classified independently as physical or psychological. The problem is that the line is so blurred that we cannot make a clear distinction, making the classification less useful than it was previously thought to be. Similarly, it is not always easy to distinguish if the person is suffering genuinely or falsifying or exaggerating the symptoms. In such cases, one must always give the benefit of doubt to the patient.

## Somatic symptom disorders

**Features:**

- One or more physical symptoms that are distressing or functionally impairing.
- Excessive or disproportionate thoughts, feelings, and behaviours about somatic symptoms.

The most important feature of somatic symptom disorders is the *somatic symptom burden*. This burden essentially defines the suffering of the patient. The burden can also be on the healthcare providers as endless consultations and tests are sought, but the physical symptoms fail to improve. Patients suffering from somatic symptom disorders might get 'cured' of one set of symptoms only to come back with another equally debilitating symptom complex.

The prevalence of somatic symptom disorder is almost 5–7% in the adult population. A person suffering from severe somatic symptom disorder will usually latch onto one symptom or a symptom complex, and no amount of evidence will convince him or her that the symptom is not serious or life-threatening. Individuals with this disorder start identifying with their symptoms and build their identity around it. This can cause severe strain on interpersonal relationships too.

People with somatic symptom disorder typically go to a primary care provider rather than psychiatrist or other mental health professional. Sometimes it can be difficult for individuals with somatic symptom disorder to understand that their concerns about their symptoms are excessive. They may continue to be fearful and worried even when they are shown evidence that they do not have a serious condition.

Let us take a classic example of this disorder. A patient comes in to see the cardiologist with chest pain. He or she describes the pain as severe, sometimes constant (intermittent but explained as constant), and points a finger to exactly where it hurts. He is convinced that it is a major cardiac issue and is terrified of being so ill. The doctor reassures the patient that this is most likely non-cardiac chest pain, but the patient is not convinced. The doctor conducts some tests including an ECG, a 2D echo, and a stress test. When all these tests reveal a normal heart function, the patient goes back, fairly convinced that it isn't angina or another severe heart ailment, but he does not feel any healthier. Soon, he starts getting severe headaches and is convinced that he has a brain tumour or something just as serious. His next visit is to a neurologist. The pattern repeats itself.

## Illness anxiety disorder

**Features:**

- Persistent, excessive thoughts and feelings about having a serious physical illness.
- Inability to be reassured.
- Minimal somatic symptoms.

The most prominent feature in illness anxiety disorder is: *The preoccupation with being ill.*

A patient suffering from Illness anxiety disorder finds it hard to stop thinking about illness despite having normal test reports and not really having somatic symptoms. The distinguishing factor here, from somatic symptom disorder, is that the patient worries about being sick or falling ill in the near future but may have no symptoms or physical complaints at that moment. This disorder is a type of anxiety disorder where the thought of falling sick plays a major role in keeping the patient preoccupied and anxious. For example, a person with illness anxiety disorder may take an antiemetic tablet, a paracetamol tablet, and some more medicines before undertaking even a short car journey, fearing the chance of getting sick (with no prior experience of actually feeling sick during a drive).

Again, people suffering from illness anxiety disorder will seek out a primary care physician, and not a mental health professional directly. The onus of making that referral lies with the physician if he or she feels that the patient is suffering emotionally despite having no identifiable disease.

## Conversion disorder (Functional neurological disorder)

**Features:**

- One or more symptoms of altered voluntary motor or sensory function.

- Evidence of incompatibility between the symptoms and recognized neurological or medical conditions.

These are a subset of psychosomatic disorders, where the symptoms are neurological and cannot be explained by a neurological disease or other medical condition. Like any other psychosomatic disorder, they are genuine and cause significant distress or problems functioning. The symptom relates to altered voluntary motor or sensory function, for example a paralysis of a limb or inability to see with one eye. It must be demonstrated to be incompatible with any known neurological or general medical condition to be diagnosed as conversion disorder.

It is no longer mandatory to document the presence of a psychological stressor or illness. The diagnosis is made irrespective of whether the person has psychological stress, frank depression or anxiety. Very important to note, is that the presence of a neurological or medical illness does not preclude the diagnosis of conversion disorder. There can be an overlap of both. For example, it is not uncommon for a person with epilepsy to also have non-epileptic attacks or a form of functional neurological disorder.

## The conditions that have been erroneously thought to be the cause of any and all psychosomatic manifestations

The conditions that we are talking about here are when the person is falsifying signs or symptoms wilfully. This is not a very common situation, though it is not rare either. The person is aware of what he or she is doing. The basic purpose is deception in order to gain something. The diagnosis can be made only if there is proof of deception or if the person confesses to it.

Persons with factitious disorder do not have any obvious gain except for a possible inner need to get medical attention. Sometimes they seem to enjoy the whole process of deceiving the medical system. It is considered a form of psychiatric disorder and classified amongst the psychosomatic disorders, though it is obviously quite different from the other psychosomatic disorders like somatic symptom disorder and illness anxiety disorder and conversion disorder where the symptoms are genuine and there is no deception. Malingering on the other hand is a personality or behavior disorder and not really considered as a disease. Here the person deceives to get some overt gain, financial compensation, or other disability benefits.

## Factitious disorder and Munchausen syndrome

This is a rare disorder accounting for around 1% of hospitalized patients, where the person deliberately falsifies physical or psychological signs or symptoms or induces injury or disease. One can suspect it in certain circumstances, but the diagnosis cannot be made unless we can prove or document the surreptitious behaviour aimed to deceive or get a confession.

Deception is clearly present, but there is no obvious external reward. It is felt that it fulfills an inner need to be seen as ill or injured, to receive affection and care, or feel like they 'belong'. For some, fooling the doctors and medical system is a game and the primary gain for them is undergoing medical tests, even invasive ones, having prolonged hospital stays, unnecessary surgeries, and being medical mysteries. They even place themselves at risk from all these procedures, but not to achieve any financial gain. Their motivations may include an adrenaline rush from undergoing medical procedures or a sense of control from deceiving healthcare professionals.

Munchausen Syndrome is a particularly extreme and chronic form of factitious disorder. There are two types of factitious disorder (and Munchausen syndrome); the first where the individual shows himself or herself to be ill, impaired or injured. ('imposed on self'). And the second, where the factitious disorder is imposed on another. This takes the deception one step ahead and the person uses someone else as a pawn (usually a child or an elderly person) to outwit the medical system. It used to be called Munchausen disorder by proxy. Here, a caregiver makes up or causes an illness or injury to a person under his or her care, a child or an elderly person. Because vulnerable people are the victims, MSBP is a form of child abuse or elder abuse. The victim is not aware of what is being done or cannot communicate the same. For example, a child whose parent has Munchausen syndrome by proxy, may be fed toxic substances to mimic food poisoning and the child may have to undergo painful tests and procedures unnecessarily.

## Malingering

This is an abnormal behavior and not really considered as an illness or disease. Like in factitious disorder, there is wilful deception; the purposeful production of falsely or grossly exaggerated physical and/or psychological symptoms. Unlike in factitious disorder, where there is no obvious external reward, in malingering the reward is obvious. It may include money, an insurance settlement, release from incarceration, or the avoidance of punishment, work, the military, or some other kind of service.

It is very important to note that these disorders are the exception and not the norm. The taboo associated with these deceitful disorders makes it very hard for doctors and patients to factor in psychological factors contributing to a disease objectively. A patient who is told that stress is the cause of his or her migraine may feel that an allegation is being made about his or her intentions. Differentiating between the genuine psychosomatic disorders and the deceitful ones, factitious and malingering, and communicating it to the patient and family is of paramount importance in lifting this taboo.

*Two terms that are very important before we navigate a book on psychosomatics are conditioned responses and validation.*

## Conditioned responses

Non-verbal cues are a very important part of all communication. While we talk casually to even a friend, we listen to what is being said, and interpret what is not being overtly said. When a friend looks away while saying something, we subconsciously register it as a false statement and might try to confirm the validity of what he or she just said. Similarly, if something we say elicits a desirable response, we are more likely to repeat what we said, even if in a subtler way.

Let us take a patient who sees a specialist with multiple symptoms. The patient is in distress, has probably had to wait a few days, at least, for his or her appointment, and then a few hours on the appointed day as well. He or she will have just a few precious minutes with the doctor before leaving with a diagnosis and a treatment plan. If this wasn't stressful enough, there will be an accompanying family member who will play a pivotal role in the healing process in the near future.

Zoom in to the actual interaction between the patient and the doctor. Let's consider the scene first. The doctor has a busy air. In fact, he looks so busy that the patient fights a fleeting sense of guilt in wasting his time. The assistant has seen the patient and the doctor has scanned the notes lying in front on the table. The patient begins by sharing some symptoms, unrelated to the disease, and the doctor, non-verbally, waves him off. Time is of the essence. The patient now mentions something else, and the doctor looks up, interested. A train of thought has begun. The patient has registered this look. He makes a subconscious note of what is an 'important' symptom. The patient relays all his symptoms one by one while noticing what the doctor pays attention to. The doctor is trying to make sense of the patient's verbal report while co-relating it to the clinical assessment. The doctor decides on the required investigations and the patient leaves with an appointment for the upcoming week with the reports.

When the patient returns, the reports are all normal or within normal limits. The doctor does a double take as this is not what was expected. With no clear diagnosis, the doctor leaves the patient with a prescription for the most pressing symptoms, for example, analgesics for pain.

The SOS medication makes the patient feel better for a while, but the symptoms persist and come back on as soon as the SOS medicines are stopped. Now, the patient seeks another opinion. This time, the patient is armed with reports and needs an answer. A diagnosis. Something. Anything to validate the illness. Anything to prove that the suffering is real. As soon as the patient meets the new doctor, he starts with the symptoms that had caught the attention of the first doctor. The original set of symptoms is 'contaminated' with knowing what the doctor probably wants to hear. This is a multi-faceted issue. Specialists from different fields might pick up and focus on different symptoms. Sometimes, the doctor might ask a question like, "Do you hear a ringing in your ear," and the patient might be more likely to tune in to any ringing sound and reply affirmatively the next time.

The patient presents the reports, and the doctor finds himself confused as the verbal description fits a particular ailment, but the reports show nothing to verify it. Again, the patient leaves with no clear diagnosis, a few 'maybes' and a prescription for SOS drugs. This cycle may repeat many times before either the patient gives up or a doctor refers him to a mental health professional. Through each cycle, the symptoms are reported with conditioned distortions. It is important to note that these conditioned distortions are learned behaviors and work on a subconscious level. They are not a conscious thought process and are not factitious or manufactured by the patient for any secondary gain.

Through all of this, the patient probably doesn't even know that his report is not complete or completely honest. His reality has slowly shifted. It might take a while for anyone to start from the beginning and pick up the missing pieces.

*One of the simplest ways to avoid this trap, as a patient, is to write down all the original symptoms before seeing a specialist. It helps in staying tuned into what was really the distress. As a doctor, the simplest way to avoid the same trap and ensure that the patient is providing a complete list of symptoms is to simply ask. Ask the patient to tell you when and how it all started. And tell them to avoid missing anything, no matter how inconsequential it may seem to the patient or any doctor they might previously have consulted. Mutual trust is paramount in such situations. The treating doctor must trust the doctor who diagnosed/treated the patient before him and trust the patient himself. This helps in gaining a strong objective perspective and also helps override the learned responses that might have been hindering a clear diagnosis.*

## Case 1

Mr A came into my office one fine Tuesday morning, having requested an urgent appointment just the previous evening. The fact that he needed to fly back to his country of work and also that his symptoms were severe, to say the least, made me agree to see him on such short notice. His symptoms included severe ptosis (heaviness and drooping of an eyelid), double vision, difficulty breathing, and malaise (a sense of being unwell). With the above list, every doctor he visited (and he did cover an astonishing number of well-known consultants) checked for Myasthenia Gravis first. His MRI was normal. All his blood tests were normal. He tested negative for Myasthenia too. When he came in, his body language was strongly suggestive of hopelessness and helplessness. He had a rather large and heavy-looking folder with details of every consultation he had sought to date for the same issue.

I asked for the file and was immediately struck by the neatness and detailing that had gone into the filing of the papers. Each section had a summary, the doctor's opinion, tests recommended, medicines prescribed, and the duration of the treatment. Next came the test reports. It was neatly arranged in chronological order and was wrapped up with the suggestions that the doctor had for further testing. The patient looked tired and seemed resigned and said in as many words that 'he was there only because the last doctor had insisted.'

The interview began and he was barely able to maintain eye contact. The patient repeated the symptoms just as they were in the file and never missed a detail, nor did he furnish any new symptoms. We decided to start with the point when he first felt that he needed medical help:

Patient: I could feel this heaviness in my eyelid sometimes. I went to a senior consultant in my town and he took down my medical history, which was surprisingly scanty as I've been healthy most of my life. He asked me if I had trouble breathing, or if I felt pain in my limbs, or if I felt weak after being active for a while etc.

Therapist: So, what all added up?

Patient: Well, I did remember feeling very tired lately. Work has been demanding, you know. But maybe it was because of this disease that the doctor suspected. Maybe it wasn't my fault.

Therapist: What else?

Patient: I have had instances when my heart starts racing and I can't breathe properly. So that added up well too.

Therapist: Did you mention the palpitations to the doctor?

Patient: No. He wanted to know about breathing. So I mentioned that.

Therapist: How did he react?

Patient: It seemed to be adding up in his mind too. He seemed to be really getting somewhere with his diagnosis.

Therapist: How did that make you feel?

Patient: He did look serious. And the tests he ordered told me something was seriously amiss.

Therapist: What happened after that?

Patient: As you can see, the reports were normal. I went to another doctor to seek a second opinion.

Therapist: And?

Patient: This time I knew what questions were coming my way, so I told him about all the symptoms I knew he would be interested in. But the normal test results left him muddled.

Therapist: And then you sought more opinions?

Patient: Yes. I have seen doctors from so many fields, I've lost count.

Therapist: Let's go back to the breathing difficulty.

Patient: What about it?

Therapist: Describe this episode for me, please. The time when you feel your heart racing and have difficulty breathing.

Patient: Um… It happens without warning. I feel like my heart will jump out of my chest. There's a strange pain. I start panting. My cheeks go warm. I'm unable to calm down.

Therapist: Has this happened at any particular time more often than others?

Patient: Um, no. I can't say a time. I feel very worked up afterwards. Sometimes it happens before I sleep. Then I end up awake, unable to really settle down.

Therapist: Has anyone in your family ever been diagnosed with an anxiety disorder? Or panic attacks?

Patient: Strange that you ask…but yes, my mother has been on anti-anxiety medicines for almost two decades now. She's dependent on those tiny pills.

The patient had developed a sense of his illness slowly, but surely, over the multitude of appointments that had been sought. What he described above are classic symptoms of panic attacks but he has never been asked to consider them because he always focused on the breathing difficulty and left the other symptoms of the panic disorder away. He did not do this intentionally. He had learnt, along the way, that certain symptoms elicited interest from the doctors while others didn't. Eventually, he started believing this distortion himself. When he looked up his symptoms online, he typed in all those that he had clubbed together in his mind and it didn't offer any clarity. He was convinced he had a major disease but the fact that there was no immediate diagnosis made him anxious. This added to the panic attacks and it became a vicious circle. The patient was inducted into therapy, while his current doctor was given regular updates. Through therapy, he came face to face with the panic that started the whole spiral and was able to step away and see it clearly. His eyelid stopped drooping and his self-confidence improved tremendously. The medicines that he was on were slowly tapered off and stopped by the doctor.

The patient remained symptom-free at 6 months and 12 months of follow up.

Having sought the patient's permission to delve deeper into the interpersonal dynamics that came into play between the patient and the various doctors, I started calling up and speaking to all the doctors that he had seen. Not very surprisingly, everyone remembered him. He was the kind of patient who always turned up on time, never showed non-compliance towards suggested treatment, was up to date with his records and, most importantly, listed his symptoms in a crisp, educated way. The doctors had all felt the same sense of confusion when the symptoms clearly pointed to a disease but the tests were all normal. He was genuinely distressed and was a likeable person. The doctors didn't want to 'write him off' and tell him that it was probably psychosomatic, although at least three of them mentioned that they had a strong feeling this could be psychosomatic. Two of the doctors also mentioned that he didn't seem like a liar, so why would this be psychosomatic and not outright organic? It would have been rude to suggest something like that.

The keywords here being *liar, written off and educated.* As a doctor, it's not easy to tell someone whom you like and trust that they need to see a psychiatrist or a psychologist. They believed that these cases belonged at the bottom of the pile. In this case, the doctors felt that they would be making an allegation about the patient by 'calling' him psychosomatic. A simple taboo, but a complicated path.

He had finally been referred for psychotherapy by a doctor who didn't know him very well personally. This helped the doctor see the nature of the complaint more objectively and didn't hinder him from suggesting mental health intervention. Sometimes the VIP syndrome can stop such a referral from taking place. When a doctor holds the patient in high esteem or knows him very well personally, he or she may be hesitant in making a referral for mental health. A clear, unbiased opinion is the simplest way forward.

## Validation

Most of the doctors I have worked with have a clear distinction in their mind about a 'real' symptom and an 'unreal' or 'imaginary' symptom. Let's take the example of pain. There is a pain scale we hear about all the time, although it is a totally subjective description of the pain. I remember once a surgeon asked a patient to rate his backache on a scale of 1 to 10. The patient didn't bat an eyelid before responding "9/10". On further questioning, he revealed that he slept comfortably at night, worked 6–7 hours a day in office, and preferred using public transport because parking was hard to find. He did mention that exercise was taking a back seat because of the severity of the pain. This description of pain and the rating of 9 left a lot to be interpreted. From a purely medical perspective, the doctor might use his discretion and clinical examination to understand the true intensity of the pain. In this sense, the rating of 9 automatically becomes a false one. In psychosomatics, however, the fact that the patient expresses his pain at a 9 is of some importance by itself. If the patient has a low pain threshold, it needs to be dealt with. If the patient does not have pain that severe but prefers to describe it like that, he or she still needs help.

Pain can be confusing even if it is not debilitating and is manageable. It is a deviation from the routine and something that the body now must either fight or surrender to. When pain is written off by any doctor, the patient can be left feeling outright miserable. Not validating someone's pain will usually not make it go away. Being unwell can and does hamper one's ability to work, whether at home or outside. This hindrance may affect not only the patient but the whole family. Understanding the pain or illness and constructing the social environment around it is hard, but of paramount importance, nonetheless.

One of the frequently used lines by well-meaning doctors is "Oh, it's nothing. It's just stress." The doctor means to say that the symptoms are being caused due to stress and there is no identifiable organic cause to them. Let's see how this may make a patient feel.

## Case 2

Mrs A was a 35-year-old IT professional. She had been married for six years and had a three year-old son. She worked half-day at office and would finish the rest of her work at home. She had a complicated pregnancy and without the help of in-laws (who live in another city) and parents, who are both ailing, she had to fend for herself with numerous visits to the doctor and frequent spells of bed rest. She has been complaining of daily chronic headaches for the past six months. A physician diagnosed the headaches as migraines and prescribed some medicines to help with the pain. The episodes did not reduced in frequency, but the intensity was a lot more now. She consulted a neurologist, afraid there was something seriously wrong with her. She was accompanied by her husband.

Mrs A: Doctor, I have severe headaches every day, and nothing that I do helps in relieving the pain.

Doctor: I can see that your physician recommended some tests?

Mrs A: Yes, doctor. Here they are. (She pulls out the MRI brain and a sheaf of papers holding the results for a comprehensive blood work up)

Doctor: Could you describe the headaches for me, please?

Mrs A: They occur during the mornings usually. One side of the head feels like it'll burst open. I want someone to just keep applying pressure to it. But I can't. I need to send my son to playschool and rush to the office.

Doctor: Is your routine hectic?

Mrs A: Yes. It can be tiring at times. But I love my work and don't want to stop.

(*The doctor, after examining the patient and looking through all the reports, came to the conclusion that there was nothing physically wrong with the patient. He also realized that overuse of medicines would be more problematic for the patient in the future. Not prescribing analgesics was the best way forward in this case)*

Doctor: Well, I have seen your reports. Don't worry. Nothing is wrong with you. It's just stress.

*The patient left the consulting room with her husband who has been quiet so far. He finally spoke up:*

Husband: I told you, it's nothing! You simply think too much. Stop worrying about small, small things and the migraine will go away. Listen to what the doctor said. It's nothing.

*The patient continued to have recurring migraines. She was, however, unable to complain or ask for help. Sometimes the headaches were debilitating. She, however, now felt responsible for them. She felt guilty about her own pain. She has now been advised psychotherapy by a friend and will start with it soon.*

This was a small example of how a doctor's intention was perfectly good, but the wrong words hampered healing. By not over-treating the pain, the doctor did the right thing. But, by using the words 'It's nothing. It's JUST stress,' the doctor didn't validate the patient's pain. He made the patient feel that stress was voluntary, and that pain caused by stress didn't need 'real' treatment.

Pain, the perception of pain, and the consequences of pain are extremely subjective entities. The fact that pain does not have a clearly defined biological cause does not make it any less real. By validating a patient's pain, the doctor makes the patient feel accepted and that opens a whole new path to healing. How would a doctor, who wishes to validate the patient's pain, then respond?

Responding to the same patient, the doctor might consider saying:

Doctor: I understand your pain. Although the reports are normal, the pain is still real. It still needs to be addressed. I believe, though, that there could be a strong element of emotional disturbances causing the pain. It will be a good idea to undertake psychotherapy to explore that angle. If, at any point, the therapist or you believe that it is worth investigating further from the physical perspective, don't hesitate to come back. We will re-examine the data and see what we can do. For now, however, I strongly recommend that you seek a therapist for at least four weeks.

The doctor is essentially saying the same thing as earlier. The difference is that in the second instance, the patient will feel validated. The patient will not feel as if she has been banished from the 'real' cure to the land of the 'mental problems'. And leaving the door open to further exploring the presence of an organic cause will leave the patient with a certain confidence that this is not the end of the treatment from the medical perspective. It will, in fact, also set the tone positively for psychotherapy.

## What are the different variations in psychosomatic ailments?

Let's broadly classify them into 3 parts:

1. Symptoms and diseases caused purely by emotional disturbances (e.g. panic attacks).

2. Symptoms that are caused by an organic disease, but which are aggravated by emotional disturbances (e.g. ulcerative colitis, diabetes, cardiac arrhythmias, etc.).

3. Emotional disturbances seen in physically well-defined ailments. This has two sub-parts:

    - Chronic ailments (e.g. diabetes, hypertension, etc.)

    - Acute ailments (e.g. An injury, a sudden cardiac event, etc.)

**1. Symptoms and diseases caused purely by emotional disturbances (e.g. panic attacks)**

## Case 3

Dr C came in alone for his first consultation. He was a renowned surgeon in a large city, and was married and had two teenage daughters. His career was better than most in his close circle and his family life was okay too. He had recently experienced severe chest pain and palpitations which made him dizzy while operating. He had fainted during one surgery and had an angiography immediately afterwards. The angiography was normal though. The fainting episode left him anxious as his job demanded 100% alertness and he was afraid now every time he entered the operation theatre. He never operated alone and always had a trusted junior by his side. The palpitations were more frequent now and his pulse during an episode would reach 110/120 bpm. His heart rate, at rest, was in the 90s. Having spoken to a few friends in the cardiology department, he was told that it was a benign arrhythmia and that he had nothing to worry about. His ECGs were normal, with just an occasional ectopic beat. He came for a session because some of his own post-operative patients had benefited from psychotherapy and he was desperately in need of a solution.

Patient: I am so sorry for having rescheduled this appointment so many times. Surgeries have been taking up more than their usual time and by the time I am done, it's usually past your working time.

Therapist: No problem, I understand. I am glad you finally made it though. So, tell me, what brings you here?

Patient: Well, as I mentioned over the phone, I have these sudden palpitations with severe chest pain. Sometimes I start hyperventilating. I had one fainting spell in my own OT. I spoke to a couple of my friends in cardiology, but they seem to think I'm fine. Some benign arrhythmia they say. My ECGs and Holter have been essentially clear, save for some ectopics. The thing is, I trust them. I am, however, very distressed with these symptoms. They are making it harder and harder for me to work normally.

Therapist: Would it be alright if I maintained a line of communication with your cardiologist? I wouldn't want to miss anything.

Patient: Sure. I did inform him that I was planning to start therapy.

Therapist: Great. Now tell me some more about these episodes. What is the nature of their intensity and frequency? Have they changed over time?

Patient: I've had sudden palpitations a few times before too. I mean before the episode in the operation theatre. A major change in my operating schedule, an OPD that promises to spill over my scheduled time, late nights, etc. have become harder to manage. The episodes have become more frequent now. Since the episode in the OT, I'm constantly on alert for the episodes. And they haven't failed me. They always turn up.

Therapist: Can you describe how you feel when an episode strikes?

Patient: I feel like my heart is racing at 200bpm, but the pulse is never faster than 120 when I check. I know my heart is skipping beats. Each time I feel like I will die. I don't know why. I always feel like I simply won't survive this episode. I start hyperventilating. I cannot sit in one place at that time. I need to keep pacing. My wife noticed this at home once and said that I kept wringing my hands.

Therapist: Have you ever woken up from your sleep with similar symptoms?

Patient: Yes, more than a couple of times.

Therapist: What made you consider psychotherapy?

Patient: I think I know somewhere deep inside that this isn't cardiac in origin. I spoke to my cardiologist about panic attacks and he said there was a possibility. I am here to see if this is, in fact, a panic attack. If it is, is there a way to cure it? I really don't want to take anxiolytics as they make me too sleepy.

Therapist: Have you taken anything for anxiety before?

Patient: Yes. I had taken alprazolam for a few months when I was a resident. I was aware that it might be habit-forming and stopped taking it soon. Thankfully, I never developed a dependence on the drug.

Therapist: There is a high probability of this being an anxiety disorder with intermittent panic attacks. The presentation is fairly clear. I understand your hesitation in starting any medication so early on, and there is a fair chance that you won't need them at all.

Patient: Right. So what next? How does this work?

Therapist: Here's what I recommend. Let us start with CBT (Cognitive Behaviour Therapy) for four weeks, keeping the diagnosis of panic attacks at the fore. We will keep your cardiologist in the loop and in case the episodes worsen or simply do not lessen, we will ask him to investigate further.

Patient: Done. Sounds good to me.

*In the case detailed above, the patient was already aware of what his problem might be. His open-minded approach and willingness to explore the realm of the mind helped him start with therapy immediately. He came face to face with deep-rooted fears and anxieties that had become a part of his personality from childhood, into adulthood. He discovered alternative ways of dealing with the identified stressors and was sincere with all his assignments. Over a period of a few weeks, he discovered that his attacks reduced in intensity and frequency. He was able to operate without fear and was soon more tuned in to his responses to anxiety as well. He learnt relaxation techniques and was his own strongest accomplice in the therapeutic process. At the end of six weeks, he visited his cardiologist and both agreed that his pulse at rest was lower, and his overall sense of wellbeing was higher. The cardiologist admitted that he did not mention panic attacks as he was afraid that the patient, being a renowned surgeon, might not have taken it too kindly and might have perceived it as a lack of confidence in his emotional strength. On a six month follow up after therapy, the patient was free of palpitations and was continuing to work with renewed vigour and confidence.*

### 2. When emotional disturbances aggravate symptoms of an organic disease

This is where almost all fields of medicine overlap with psychosomatics. As is discussed in the other chapters ahead, various physical symptoms are clearly worsened by emotional distress, leading to overmedication at times, and sometimes even leading to unnecessary investigations.

## Case 4

Mrs L had been suffering from rheumatoid arthritis since six years. She regularly visited her rheumatologist and was on a set regime of medicines. She had a preteen daughter and worked from home. The doctor had noticed that every three months or so, she reported aggravated symptoms and needed a slight change in medication to bring relief. During these phases of aggravation, she would report distressing symptoms and would be convinced her medicines had stopped working. Her blood tests would confirm a slight change in parameters (although not as dramatic as her perception of the change). After a few months, she reported severe migraines and was seen by a neurologist. She was then referred for psychotherapy to try and learn some coping mechanisms as overuse of medicines would have had an undesirable long-term impact.

She was hesitant to try therapy at first. To her, therapy was a land of emotional mumbo-jumbo and she felt that she would be labelled by her family and peers. On the behest of the neurologist though, she came for one session, telling herself that she would only come for one session. As rapport was established, she visibly relaxed and realized that this was not an attempt to write off her physical symptoms, but, in fact, an attempt to deal with the symptoms from a physical as well as emotional perspective. Through the course of therapy, a pattern emerged. The patient's daughter was going through puberty and had recently had some anger management issues. She was also lagging behind in her academic performance. Whenever a school exam came up, she would throw tantrums and refuse to listen to her parents or teachers. This stress would engulf everyone at home for as long as the exams lasted. Soon, her mother started preempting the anxiety and the days before the exams would be fraught with stress. This was leading to the variation she was experiencing in her symptoms. It was also the cause of her debilitating migraines. As the pattern became evident, acceptance followed. She learnt through psychoeducation that her stress was having severe physical ramifications on her body and that it was avoidable to a great extent. She learnt biofeedback techniques, relaxation methods, and also alternative ways of addressing the stressors that she could not control. She soon noticed that her symptoms stopped getting worse around exam time and she felt more in control and was able to stay healthy on the same doses of medicines that the rheumatologist had earlier prescribed. Her migraines also reduced in intensity and frequency and she reported a better quality of life.

## 3. Diseases where the cause of the ailment is purely organic, and where the nature of the disease causes emotional turmoil, in turn having an effect on the healing process

These can be further classified as:

a. Acute

b. Chronic

**Acute:**

An acute ailment could be the sudden onset of a disease or an injury. It is usually severe, but is short term and has a clear starting and ending point. A dengue fever, for example, is a disease that is caused by a specific agent, needs treatment, and eventually resolves. A fractured hand after a fall is also an example of an acute ailment. The suddenness of the ailment can have an impact on the mind and the patient might feel helpless and out of control. Keeping calm emotionally during any acute disease or injury aids quicker recovery and lowers the need for analgesics. Usually, in this case, a mental health professional is not needed. The treating doctor can establish a calm state of mind in the patient through clear explanations of the problem and a good bedside manner.

**Chronic:**

Let's look at one of the most common chronic diseases: diabetes mellitus. A diagnosis of diabetes comes with its own dictums: a change in food habits, a change in lifestyle, a close watch on blood sugar levels, and daily medication. For someone who may not have experienced any chronic ailment before receiving this diagnosis, it can be a rather scary prospect.

What makes matters worse is the availability of endless 'cures', some offered by quacks, some by others in non-medical fields. People are tempted to follow the easier way out, but eventually learn that they didn't really beat their disease. Acceptance is the most important in any chronic illness, as is the trust in the doctor providing the treatment. Mild to moderate depression is commonly seen in patients suffering from diabetes. It is sometimes brought on by the disease itself, sometimes by other factors. It is extremely essential to recognize and deal with emotional disturbances to improve the outcome of the management of the disease.

*Therapy goals are different for all three segments of illness. In the first set, where the physical symptoms are caused purely by the mind, psychotherapy can achieve complete recovery. Patients do well on follow-ups and if there is a recurrence of symptoms, re-initiating therapy is known to be helpful. In the second set, where a person's emotional responses aggravate existing organic symptoms, like in IBS, psychotherapy can achieve fair symptomatic control. Patients also report better quality of life despite occasional symptoms and lead a healthier lifestyle. In the third set, psychotherapy helps a patient come to terms with the chronic nature of their disease. Patients learn to look at their irrational beliefs and set new, practical goals for the medical treatment plan. Therapy is known to increase compliance and reduce risky behaviour with respect to a patient's health.*

# Chapter 2

# Pain: A Mind Game

Pain is the most common symptom bringing one to a doctor. The cause of the pain may not be obvious. Nonetheless it can be highly debilitating. There is a strong two-way correlation between emotional distress and pain with each being able to influence and aggravate the other.

The word pain itself originally meant suffering inflicted as a punishment for an offence. To this day, we largely look at pain as undesirable. Actually pain is a warning and protective system, essential for our well-being and survival. Sometimes, though, this system overreacts and leads to unnecessary or excessive pain.

We instinctively assume that pain in some part of our body indicates an ongoing injury there. In chronic pain, this may not be true at all, and the cause may lie far away, in a nerve or in the brain. Emotions have a huge role in chronic pain and may be disregarded while attention gets wrongly focused on some minor aberration in the painful area. Just because pain is severe or disabling does not mean the cause may not be psychological. The new realization is that pain may not be warning us of tissue injury but may be more of a signal that the brain feels is a threat, either physical or emotional.

Even in situations where the mind is playing an elaborate role in the experience of pain, it is wrong to expect the unfortunate sufferer to simply summon up willpower and become pain-free. Chronic pain requires a sensitive multi-pronged approach.

## Definition

The International Association for the Study of Pain defines pain as an *unpleasant sensory and emotional experience associated with actual or potential tissue damage or described in terms of such damage.*

All the above points are important; the unpleasantness of pain is what drives us to do something about it; the fact that it is also an emotion and not just a sensation reminds us to pay attention to the emotional state; it involves threat or potential injury and hence the physical aspect is crucial too. When we accept that pain is subjective, it means that if a person says he feels pain, we must accept it as true, even if we do not find any evidence of disease to explain the pain.

## Pain and tissue damage

You step on a thorn, it pierces your skin, you feel pain in the toe, and you immediately move your foot away and remove the thorn. In acute situations, pain protects us from further injury and is directly proportional to the amount of local injury.

This is often not so in chronic pain, where pain can be grossly out of proportion to the injury. In a curious condition called phantom limb pain, even a non-existent amputated limb, may keep paining.

Conversely, pain may be absent despite significant injury. This may happen because some organs like the brain, liver, or kidney do not have sensors for pain, or nerves carrying pain may be damaged by diseases like diabetes or leprosy. Persons with a faulty pain system are actually cursed with repeated and unrealized injuries.

The brain can decide whether it wants to pay attention to the pain, amplify it, turn it down, or shut it down totally. We all have heard stories where despite a bullet wound, a soldier feels pain only hours later when the battle is over. This stress induced analgesia is very important for survival as we shall see later.

Pain is very subjective and for various reasons, two persons may have quite different pain responses to the same injury.

## Understanding the purpose of pain

Pain has traditionally been thought to be a system warning us of tissue injury. Let us see how pain evolved in man from a primitive self-preservation instinct to a threat detection system.

Even the single-celled amoeba detects danger and moves away from it. As animals evolved, they developed better ways of detecting and responding to damage and danger. The addition of emotion to pain, in higher animals, made it more effective, in that they moved away faster,

Man being a thinking animal took it a step further. Not only does man sense and feel pain but he also thinks about it, compares it with the past, stores away the memory for the future, plans how to avoid it but also thinks about the significance or meaning of the pain.

In fact, our brain does not wait for tissue injury to happen; even the possibility of damage or a perceived threat evokes pain. Pain is the brain's assessment and opinion of the situation, with the express purpose of protecting us. Conversely, if the brain feels no danger, the pain will not be felt despite tissue damage.

Let us now also look at what pain is trying to protect. We said that the purpose of pain is to protect us; but it is protecting not just our body, but also our emotional self and mind, or the person in us, so to say. In earlier times, we did not try to distinguish between pain of the mind and emotional self, and pain of the body. Even today we say, "You are such a pain" or "You hurt me" or "You stabbed me in the back"; "His words pierced my heart"; "Like a crushing burden on my shoulders"; "This news came to me as a big blow," and so on. Western science and dualistic thinking went on to separate pain of the body from pain of the mind. Real pain was the one that arose in the body and had some demonstrable abnormality or explanation. This was contrasted with imaginary pain arising in the mind, called psychological pain. Persons with real pain got sympathy and validation, while those with psychological pain were treated as if they were exaggerating the pain or were in some way emotionally weak. Only real pain needed to be managed by a medical doctor, while psychological pain was for psychiatrists or counsellors to manage. This psychological pain was labelled as suffering, anguish or torment in order to distinguish it from 'real pain'.

We now know that dualistic thinking is a fallacy and just as the mind and body are two aspects of the same person, there is no real difference between the two kinds of pain. In fact, functional MRI shows similar patterns of activity in the brain, whether the person has physical pain, psychological pain, or even feels empathy on seeing someone else in pain. Even the definition of pain clearly accepts that it is subjective.

## How do we feel pain?

Rene Descartes, the influential thinker of Dualistic philosophy, looked at pain as a simple one-way signaling system informing the brain about tissue injury. We now know that it is much more complex than that. Let us see what happens when one stubs their toe against a rock. We used to think that the injured toe sends a telegram like message to the brain, " Injury is happening at the toe" and then the brain reacts to it. This is not the whole truth. The brain is much more sophisticated. It is not passively receiving information from the toe and responding to it. It decides which messages will be allowed to reach awareness, whether to block them totally or allow them through or even whether to sort of roll out the red carpet for them and ignore everything else.

Special sensors at the periphery, called nociceptors, detect tissue damage, and send electrical messages to the brain. The messages are carried by nerves first to the spinal cord, where the neurons behave like a gate, either blocking or allowing them to go ahead. Acupuncture, rubbing the painful part or applying a balm work, in a way by crowding out the pain signals at the gate. More importantly, the brain can open or close the gate at will. For example, during a battle, a closed gate works better than most painkillers and the soldier feels no pain. The opposite situation happens in chronic pain where sensitization makes even simple touch feel painful.

Pain messages go to various regions of the brain; a fast pathway tells us immediately where it is hurting and our foot gets pulled away almost automatically. Simultaneously a slower pathway informs the emotional areas of the brain and, a few seconds later, we get the unpleasant feeling of pain which motivates us to take corrective action. The memory and planning areas of the brain also store away this information for the future.

It is very important to understand that like all other perceptions and feelings, pain is an opinion of the brain and is modified by what the brain knows, expects, fears, and thinks. So the brain takes in all the available information, uses its memory and other capacities and makes an assessment. Only if the brain concludes that there is a threat or danger, does it allow the person to feel pain. During a battle, the brain may decide that it is more dangerous to stop fighting and so it produces morphine-like chemicals called endorphins to block the pain till the battle is over. Endorphins act at multiple levels; at the spinal gate they block the pain messages, and in the brain, they reduce the emotional response to pain. All this allows the person to run away or fight when attacked, rather than get immobilized. On the other hand, since pain is more of a threat signal, the more insecure and anxious the brain feels, the more the pain.

## The types of pain

There are three types of pain, one with actual tissue injury, one with nerve dysfunction and one without any ostensible reason.

The first one with actual tissue injury is called nociceptive pain, the main one in acute situations.

The second is neuropathic pain, where the pain system itself malfunctions and sends wrong messages to the brain, misinforming it of tissue injury, when there is none. This leads to chronic pain in nerve disorders like diabetic neuropathy or sciatica.

The third type of pain is called chronic primary pain and is even more complex. There is no tissue damage, no nerve dysfunction, and yet the person feels pain. The brain itself seems to create the sensation of pain due to a complex interplay of biological, psychological, and social factors. Complex regional pain syndrome, fibromyalgia, chronic migraine, and irritable bowel syndrome belong to this category.

## Sensitization

Our brain is excellent at learning anything with practice by developing and enhancing connections and information exchange between neurons. Unfortunately, it also learns how to feel more pain. This process called sensitization becomes very important in chronic pain.

Even relatively primitive animals like flies develop increased overall sensitivity to pain after any significant injury. The purpose is to protect the animal from further injury. Central sensitization is particularly common in chronic pain disorders. Sensitization leads to more pain signals reaching the brain, along with increased brain sensitivity as the brain changes itself. The pain now spreads out, lasts longer, and feels more severe. Even simple touch or small movements may cause pain. The basic defect in primary pain disorders might be sensitization at the level of the brain.

People differ greatly in their pain response to the same injury; sensitization may differ from person to person, depending on genetic backgrounds, lifestyle, and life events. Sensitization is aggravated by anticipating pain, by feeling threatened or worried. The more you worry about what might be the cause of pain or what it could lead to, the worse the pain may feel. On the other hand, being overall physically fit, having healthy habits, and being happier, relaxed, and secure reduces sensitization. Interestingly, opioid analgesics may promote sensitization and so are not a good idea for treating chronic pain.

## Managing chronic pain

Chronic pain has more to do with central sensitization than with local tissue injury, and so, rather than focusing on the site of pain, it is often worth paying attention to the person's lifestyle and emotional state.

The patient and family need to understand the role of emotions and central sensitization in chronic pain and how we can reduce pain by addressing these. Then they can appreciate and accept general measures like fitness, exercise, good sleep, healthy habits and lifestyle, and techniques like hypnosis, cognitive behavior therapy and meditation.

Avoiding movement is desirable in the early stages for proper healing, like a plaster cast for a fracture. But once healing has begun, graded movement is helpful. At this stage, fear of movement due to pain is counterproductive. It is important to explore the right amount and type of activity under the supervision of the doctor or therapist.

Chronic pain itself also leads to various secondary psychological disorders like anxiety and depression, which may further worsen the pain. Psychological therapy like CBT may be helpful and some persons may benefit from drug therapy. In general, one should avoid drugs, including painkillers and anti-epileptic drugs, though acupuncture and antidepressants have been shown to be useful in some situations.

## Summary

Chronic pain affects the person as a whole and has more to do with the mind and the emotional state of the person than with tissue damage.

A threatened brain develops more sensitization and more pain, and so, making the person feel less worried and secure helps. Learning to be fit, healthy, and happy also goes a long way in reducing chronic pain.

It is important to emphasize that all pain is real, and needs empathy as well as medical and physical treatment.

## Case 1

A pleasant and young lady came to me almost 10 years ago for persistent pain in her hand. She had injured her left wrist in a car accident and had pain and numbness in the hand. She was given medicines, to begin with, but as the pain did not settle down, she underwent release of the nerve going to her thumb. She continued to experience pain, numbness, swelling as well as redness of the hand intermittently, despite various treatments including physiotherapy, splinting, wax baths, and many drugs.

A hand surgeon did another surgery and removed a ganglion from the wrist and also released what he felt was nerve compression. As this surgery did not work, he operated on the nerve, in an attempt to block the pain messages to the spinal cord. This provided some relief but did not provide complete relief from occasional painful flareups. During these episodes, the wrist would be visibly inflamed and red.

I found her pain out of proportion to the local tissue and nerve damage. She was obviously suffering, but I sensed something else was at play rather than only local damage. As I got to know her better, I realized she was expecting too much from herself, trying to excel on many fronts simultaneously, as a wife, a daughter-in-law, a mother, a professional, and also at her own hobbies. She was highly intelligent, well-read, and keen to understand what was happening. She did not like to compromise on any front.

I pointed out to her that what she had was what we call complex regional pain syndrome which gets triggered by an initial injury but later on often gets sustained and aggravated by various emotional and social factors. We saw clearly how her emotional state could affect her hand and cause it to even become red and swollen.

Over the last few years, the pain gradually settled down with some relapses, when under great emotional or physical stress.

## Case 2

Two years ago, after an attack of sciatica due to a slipped disc, I gained several insights about radicular pain from the perspective of not just a doctor, but a patient too.

For one, unlike what I had been taught all along, the pain was not radiating along the nerve from the back to the leg; nor was it sharp and shooting. In fact, it was a very characterless and non-descript pain, once in the buttock region, another day in the thigh and sometimes in the leg. If I had not known better, I would have diagnosed it as a musculoskeletal pain rather than a nerve pain.

The second insight was realizing how much pain can disturb one emotionally and mentally and make one irrational. My knowledge told me that sciatica pain would settle down within a few weeks with rest and physiotherapy and surgery had no role or advantage. But every few days, as the pain recurred, I would find myself getting frustrated and anxious, and even toying with the idea of some surgery to get relief.

The relation of pain to mood and stress levels was driven home in a striking way. I had restarted work once the pain had reduced. On some days, the pain would get inexplicably worse and would get me to worry. I would often wonder whether the disk had gotten prolapsed again. Only later did I realize the correlation of these fluctuations with my own stress levels. If I had an emotionally demanding or stressful day, the pain would worsen. The worsening pain would pull me further down emotionally. It was indeed a spiral. This ordeal made me more sensitive towards the pain my patients were experiencing. I now knew how exhausting pain could be, how vague that exhaustion could sound, and yet, how real and debilitating it all could be.

## Case 3

A pleasant 64 year old gentleman came recently and reported being unwell for the past six months. He had seen me eight years ago for migraine, had improved and was alright for the last few years. He was diabetic and hypertensive with poor cardiac function. But in the last six months, his cardiac function had worsened, and he could not sleep lying down flat in bed due to breathlessness and had a constant feeling of pressure over his chest.

Strangely, in the last six months, he also started getting multiple other aches and pains, each with their own medical explanations; pain in the shoulders was attributed to frozen shoulder and pain in the heel to a bony spur. His symptoms continued despite seeing multiple doctors. Quite sheepishly he confessed that there was no point in his body which was not paining.

Gradually as he opened up, it came to light that ever since the Covid pandemic broke out and a lockdown was declared in Pune, he started to worry about his heart condition even more and was terrified of not being able to find a hospital bed available in case of an emergency. We explained to him that all his new aches and pains were not due to multiple new problems, but an overall dialing up of pain perception by his brain due to the anxiety and insecurity. With reassurance by the cardiologist, psychologist and the neurologist and medicines to reduce his anxiety, he gradually started feeling better.

# Chapter 3
# Headache: The Aching Mind

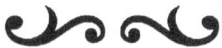

"Daddy, my mind is paining," said my three-year-old daughter to me years ago. At that time, I remember smiling at what I thought was her naivety and telling her that it is the brain which pains and not the mind. But, today, after almost 30 years, and after treating thousands of patients, I have come to accept that she was, at least, as right as me. Headache arises as much from the mind as from the brain, and to treat migraine effectively, you need to pay attention to both.

This artificial separation of the mind from the body and the brain was spearheaded by Rene Descartes and later Western thinkers. For thousands of years, ancient wisdom had viewed the whole person, recognizing the intertwined nature of the mind and body. Many systems of medicine like Ayurveda, Homeopathy, Tibetan and Chinese medicine consider the mind, body and spirit as one. Dualistic thinking separated the physical from the non-physical, the objective and external like the sciences from the subjective and internal like the arts, and the brain (and body) from the mind. The brain like the body was considered as a material substance that could be touched, seen, and visualized in life, while the mind could be studied only by introspection, or indirectly by making a judgement about how another person thought or felt. Medicine focused on what could be documented or observed. This later led to a barrier coming up between neuroscientists, who studied the brain, and psychologists, who probed the mind, between neurological disorders of the brain and psychiatric disorders of the mind. This influence of dualistic thinking has been so powerful that many lay persons, as well as doctors, still consider neurological or organic disorders 'more real' than psychiatric or functional disorders.

We know better now and consider the mind and the brain to be different and yet not separate. They are aspects of the same person, in some ways, akin to the hardware and software components of a computer. It is not the brain alone which is involved in thinking; instead, there is evidence to suggest that the whole body, including the gut, are involved in thinking and feeling. The brain and mind can affect each other; for example, brain damage can affect a person's thinking, while learning a new skill changes the brain; specific areas of the brain increase in size or sprout new connections.

I feel we have focused mainly on the brain and not given the mind its due place in the patient with migraine and similar headaches.

## Primary headaches

Headache is among the top causes of disability across the world, most of them being primary headaches; conditions, where the person tends to get headaches, but has no abnormal finding on examination or testing. Secondary headaches, due to a demonstrable disease like a brain tumour, acute sinusitis or glaucoma are by far the exception. The commonest primary headaches are tension type headache and migraine. Half of the world's population will get tension type headache sometime in their lifetime and another 10 percent will have migraine. Their diagnosis is based on the history or the description of the headache and matching it to certain criteria, formulated by a group of experts. The examination and all tests are normal in both and so no test distinguishes between them. Some headaches can look somewhat like migraine and somewhat like tension type headache or some persons can have headaches which look like migraine one day and tension type headache on another day. The name matters in many ways though. When they call it tension type headache, doctors rightly focus their attention on tension, stress, and lifestyle. But once a headache is called migraine, it almost becomes hallowed and evokes much more interest in treatment as well as research. Now tension, stress and lifestyle are mentioned only in passing. The focus changes to a search for some basic defect in migraine, with the expectation that soon there will be a cure for migraine; doctors are willing, nay, quite keen to try exotic and expensive drugs, inject medicines into the scalp, give electrical or magnetic pulses to the brain and so on.

Imagine the difference the name makes to patients. Once awarded the label of migraine, they gain the treating doctor's interest, plus everyone's sympathy and validation. The doctor may declare, "You have Migraine. We shall start a course of treatment for a few months, and you should soon feel better." These lucky patients can blame their genes and proudly bandy the diagnosis in social conversations: "You know, I couldn't come that day for work as I got hit by my migraine". The unfortunate person who is labelled tension type headache is made to feel almost ashamed, as if they are boring and wasting time of the treating doctor who may say in a perfunctory and almost disdainful manner "It's nothing, just tension headache. Relax and try not to get stressed out so much." This patient is left unhappy and dissatisfied and may hide or deny the diagnosis and may seek another doctor. Patients are quite proud to tell me they have been diagnosed to have migraine, but this never happens with tension type headache. Funnily enough, neurologists label their own headaches as migraine and almost never as tension type headache.

The basic difference seems to me, that tension type headache is considered functional, attributed to the mind and the responsibility is on patients, their actions, thoughts, or behavior, while migraine is considered organic, attributed to the brain; and is blamed on bad luck or bad genes. I personally see both as shades of grey of the same primary headache disorder, and I do not find that the approach to management differs much. So, I shall talk of both as migraine henceforth.

Many who have migraine wrongly attribute their headaches to sinus disease, blood pressure, acidity, spondylosis, or a minor refractory error, and focus their attention on avoiding or correcting these. The misdiagnosis correlates with the triggers. For example, the 'sinus person' has frontal headaches after cold beverages or exposure to air-conditioned rooms, the 'acidity' one may get a headache on missing meals, or having excess tea, or oily or sour or spicy food; and 'spondylosis' may lead to pain in the neck and at the back of the head on working in the kitchen or on a laptop. Interestingly, these patterns run in families. A person with a headache due to acidity often has a parent with similar acidity.

## Allostasis, stress and migraine

A thermostat has the function of maintaining the temperature in your refrigerator around a set point; for example, when the temperature falls below the set level, it reduces cooling, and the temperature goes up; when it gets too hot, it sets into motion cooling to bring down the temperature towards the set level. A primitive area of the brain called the hypothalamus acts similarly for hundreds of internal body parameters, like body temperature, blood pressure, and blood sugar. We used to think that this process called homeostasis was how our internal environment or mileu interior was kept within the tight range needed for our health and survival.

Homeostasis evolved millions of years ago in the primitive nervous systems of worms. Our brains are, of course, much more sophisticated and experts now believe our health depends on a more intelligent and efficient process called allostasis and not homeostasis. Allostasis is predictive unlike homeostasis, which is reactive and kicks in only after things go out of range. In short, our brain does not wait to make corrections after change has happened; it intelligently predicts what is likely to happen and takes preemptive action. For example, we feel hunger much before our blood sugar level falls and feel satiated much before our blood sugar goes up. We see gathering dark clouds and pick up an umbrella. We don't give rain a chance to soak us.

Every change or threat of change is a task for the brain. The brain is the central organ of stress, assessing and dealing with threats, constantly making computations and decisions. All this hard work needs energy. It stands to reason that excessive stress or allostatic overload would end up troubling the brain and migraine is what happens when the brain gets troubled. There is considerable evidence to implicate the hypothalamus in migraine. Migraine may be the price our brain pays for demand exceeding capacity. The most common trigger of migraine is, in fact, stress or a sudden letdown of stress. Perceived stress has already been shown to predict a migraine. In fact, I would not be surprised, if we soon get an app on our phone to give a forecast about a migraine attack based on how we say the day has been. The fact that migraine often holds out till the stressful event gets over, makes one wonder whether the brain summons up whatever energy reserves it has, to tide over the stress and only later allows the headache to kick in, when the energy is exhausted.

Stress can be physical, emotional, or mental; inadequate sleep, missing mealtimes, illness in the family, upcoming exams, or job interviews, shifting house, overwork at the job or home, interpersonal issues, retirement, financial worries to name a few. What is stressful varies from person to person and even in the same person from time to time. I once had a doctor friend narrate to me how a bad migraine was triggered by his driving down to a nearby city to pick up his sister-in-law at the airport. He confessed quite innocently, that two months ago, when he had driven to the same airport to pick up his own brother, he did not get a headache. I have the impression, after seeing thousands of headaches, that an enjoyable activity is less likely to trigger a headache. But when one feels compelled to do the same activity it becomes stressful. I wonder, if just deciding to accept things or trying to like them, might make them less stressful.

Stressors and triggers somehow trigger chemical and electrical changes in the brain called spreading depression, which is one of the first steps in the migraine attack.

## Could migraine have any purpose?

Like other pains, I believe migraine is also a beneficial protective mechanism that every brain is capable of; the tendency is essentially inherited and varies from person to person. It can be looked upon as a useful strategy and defense mechanism of the brain in dealing with excessive stress and it serves to restore the energy balance and rejuvenate the fatigued and overworked brain. Various abnormalities have been shown in the migraine brain just before an attack, which get corrected after the attack. Of course, in some unfortunate persons, it can become excessive and troublesome by itself.

Migraine is not something man has invented. As other animals cannot tell us about their headache, we must infer it from their behavior and look for equivalents of migraine. Let us look at how migraine may have evolved over millions of years by studying animal behavior, and coping strategies when responding to threats.

When faced with a threat, even one-celled primitive amoeba-like organisms show a withdrawal response. Higher animals evolved more nuanced responses. One response is active, the fight or flight response while the other response is passive or 'playing possum', where the animal behaves as if it is dead, in order to fool a predator. When faced with infection or other disease, an animal often exhibits what is called *sickness behaviour*, which is like a milder form of 'playing dead'; the animal withdraws, reduces activity, and spends more time resting or sleeping; it basically conserves its energy and recovers. But this is exactly what a migraine attack does for you.

A migraine attack forces you to take rest and allows you to get rejuvenated, as if returning from a 'mini-hibernation'. There is some suggestion that having migraine gives the person an evolutionary survival advantage and this may be the reason migraine remains such a common disorder all over the world.

It seems reasonable that if you do not allow a buildup of this energy mismatch, by treating your brain with tender loving care and respect, by regular and adequate sleep, meals and exercise, and enjoyable relaxation activities, the brain may no longer need headaches and you could prevent migraine.

## How do I explain migraine to patients?

I tell patients that like overused muscles, the head aches when you trouble it excessively. Some people can tolerate a late meal or lack of sleep and not get a headache. But migraineurs inherit a more sensitive brain, often from one or both parents. Their brains are not able to adapt to loud noises or stressors and so they get headache more easily than others. One late night, one missed meal, and it may strike.

I explain to them in simple terms how migraine can be protective or even beneficial and arise from demands outstripping capacity. I tell them to look upon it as an alarm, which is alerting them and giving them the opportunity to take corrective steps before something more serious happens. I may give an analogy of the whistle of a pressure cooker; it allows the person to literally let off steam and reduce the load on the brain. Sometimes I may tell them it behaves like a speed governor or speed breaker on the road, it limits multitasking and overworking.

I tell them how, as a migraineur, I know that occasional headaches are to be expected. But frequent headaches means that some issue needs to be sorted out. Rather than a disease to be cured, migraine needs to be understood as a lifelong tendency, which needs learning to live with and handling appropriately.

Once I establish this, we try to explore what could be causing the present trouble or excessive demands, what might have happened or changed in their life recently; a new job, exams coming up, getting married recently, or a newborn baby spoiling his/her sleep, or a difficult new boss, or deadlines at work. Patients often deny tension or stress, but easily accept the more acceptable and neutral word *hectic*.

In fact, I tell them to learn to prepare for aggravation in various stages of their lives, like exams, college admissions, job hunting, marriage, becoming a parent, empty nest syndrome, menopause, retirement, losing a loved one, and so on. I do tell them that it generally settles down in most people with age, maybe as they accumulate wisdom of handling life's problems and issues.

## How do I manage migraine?

Even when the examination and scan come normal, I continue to listen with genuine interest; reassure the patient, validate their suffering and let them know that I believe their symptoms are real. This establishes rapport and allows me to become a healer, an adviser to treat the mind as well as the brain.

I explain the biopsychosocial model of migraine in simple terms; I tell them how the genetic predisposition is the biological abnormality and how that interacts with their psychological and social stressors to lead to the headaches. Once I rule out additional biological aggravators, I help the patients to explore psychosocial aspects of their life. This often gives them an insight into their life and kickstarts a corrective process which often leads to the headaches reducing without much drug therapy. I tell them that I shall prescribe drugs for a few months to give them time to sort out the present problems. I tell them to not expect a cure, but a strategy and skills to handle their migraine tendency and cope with it better in the future. I explain how it helps to increase *brain reserves* by adopting a healthy lifestyle with regular sleep, meals, and exercise, meditation or other relaxation activities.

I always enquire about the commonly associated functional illnesses, like irritable bowel syndrome, chronic backache, neck pain, sleep disorders, anxiety and depression and address them as well, explaining their interrelation.

The pandemic has clearly resulted in the worsening of migraine in many patients and underscored the relation of migraine to overall stress. Sleep, daily routines and exercise schedules have been disrupted, anxiety levels and insecurity have gone up, work has increased on various fronts. This has been compounded by fear and difficulty in consulting their doctors.

## *Concluding Remarks*

I believe migraine, like all pain, basically serves a protective function. It serves to protect the brain as well as the mind. Like with the other functional disorders, it is crucial to treat the person.

Stress interacts with the sensitive migraine brain to cause headaches, and so, attention must be directed to the biological issues as well as the psycho-social ones. We need to look upstream, on why the brain gets the migraine attacks, be it lifestyle, stress, hormones, or other issues. Drugs like triptans, and even the new CGRP blockers work downstream, on ameliorating or blocking the effects. Like my daughter had said, it is the mind paining and not just the brain.

## Case 1

An anxious couple once got their son to me for his frequent headaches. The parents had an IT job and had shifted to Pune four months ago. Soon afterwards, their nine-year-old son started getting headaches. Initially, he would come back home and complain of headache, later he started returning home from school. For the last two weeks, he used to get severe headaches with vomiting, sometimes in the morning, preventing him from going to school. His examination and MRI were normal, and he had not responded to drugs commonly used for childhood migraine.

I asked the child what he did in the day, now that he was not going to school. He told me, quite languidly, that he gets out of bed, around 10 a.m. and then would watch television, play some games on the computer or the phone. The boy looked quite comfortable and not in any major distress and I had the feeling he seemed to be enjoying his 'holidays'. I asked the child to wait outside and explained to his anxious parents that there was no structural problem with the brain. Something was troubling the child and I wondered if he was somehow not happy going to the new school. The parents vehemently denied this and said that, in fact, the child was very keen to go to school and every night would cry and plan to go to school the next day and even keep his bag packed. But, come morning, the headache would arrive before the school bus. I explained to the parents, that it was possible that one part of his mind did sincerely want to go to school but subconsciously, his mind was not happy and missing the old one. Finally, the parents relented and met the school counsellor and the class teacher. Soon the child settled down, made new friends, and started enjoying the new school, and his headaches stopped.

A common situation in children is frequent headaches preventing them from going to school or extra tuition, or headaches before an exam. The ones who suffer are often those who fail or those who are toppers; the average ones are quite relaxed as they don't feel stressed out.

## *Case 2*

A 26-year-old girl came for frequent headaches in the last three years. The headaches were typically like migraine; several specialists had seen her, done several scans and tried various drugs. She gained a lot of weight, while the headaches continued unabated.

I have a rough checklist in my mind for migraines at various ages; at this age, the usual problems I find are studies, career, job, or relationship/marriage issues. After graduating with a gold medal in Bachelor of Computer Application, for the last three years, she was trying to get selected in the UPSC, a competitive exam to get a civil service post. It turned out that this was her father's dying wish, before he passed away three years ago. Not only was she depressed with the untimely loss of her father but was getting extremely stressed trying to clear the UPSC exam. She even had suicidal thoughts and needed psychiatric help to recover.

## Case 3

A 32-year-old man came to me accompanied by his father. He had rare headaches in the past. But from 2016, he had started getting headaches once or even twice a week. They were sometimes accompanied by a sensation of losing balance and he would have to stand and hold on for support for a minute or so. Now, for the last one week, he was getting headache and dizziness every day.

He had consulted several doctors, got MRI done thrice and tried many drugs for migraine and vertigo. His tests were all normal and suggested the possibility of migraine both as the cause of his headaches and the imbalance.

Initially, they denied any cause for stress or overwork. I said to them, "We need to find out why the headaches and dizziness have worsened. With my normal examination and the normal MRIs, I feel something must be troubling his brain. Is there any change in his routine, overwork or some stress.?" The son shook his head, but after a minute of thinking, wondered out aloud, if it might be related to the marital stress that his son was facing. On asking for details, it turned out that he got married in 2014 but had never really got along with his wife. This had culminated in a divorce case, which was to come up for hearing in two days.

To an observer, it seems obvious that so much marital stress and an upcoming divorce hearing would cause headaches. But, inexplicably, patients do not put two and two together or underplay the stress and try to look for other causes.

Counselling and temporary psychiatric help solved the young man's problem and helped him get through the divorce. His headaches and dizziness settled down gradually with that.

## Jobs and headache

Everything about a job can cause headaches, finding one, losing one, getting a promotion, having a difficult boss, getting a new boss, facing deadlines and targets, and coworkers falling ill. Retirement is a difficult time for many.

## *Case 4*

Around five years ago, a 30-year-old pleasant young lady came to see me. She has a headache and sudden forgetfulness for one day, which started after she came back from cycling out in the sun. She did have occasional migraine headaches once or twice in a month for the last 10 years. She had a history of not being able to sleep well for the last few years and a tendency to get worked up about her children. But this time, the headache was a little more severe than her usual ones and strangely, she could not remember having gone out cycling.

Her family and the family doctor attributed her headache to cycling in the hot sun.

I examined her and found no neurological abnormality and felt this was a routine migraine attack, except for the memory problem. So, I insisted on getting an MRI brain done. Everyone was taken aback when her MRI showed a large vascular malformation in the brain.

There was an abnormal tangle of blood vessels inside her brain, which could burst at any time.

Such cases are rare but can make the doctor overcautious in dealing with every headache or every medically unexplained symptom. Missing this headache and attributing it to stress would have been a disaster for both the patient as well as the doctor. This may be a reason why doctors are hesitant to label something as functional. But this often leads to over investigation and missing the appropriate management of the underlying psycho-social issues. It is very important to realize that these cases are the exceptions, not the norm. In most other cases, stress would have been a very likely cause of a severe migraine.

When it comes to the practice of neurology, in particular headache, the neurologist has to tread a fine line. Just considering every medically unexplained symptom to be functional is not right and can be downright dangerous. On the other hand, only finding that there is some emotional disturbance or stressor should not lead you to think that the symptoms are functional. It has to be a positive diagnosis based on the lack on medical explanation plus the pattern of illness. Missing an organic disorder like an AVM or a brain tumour can have serious ramifications. Investigations and tests are, of course, necessary but one has to draw the line somewhere and not keep on repeating tests endlessly. Also one has to take into consideration the opinion of the mental health specialist and the response to psychological therapy. A joint management approach, with the neurologist and the psychologist is the safest and most effective approach.

# CHAPTER 4
# Gastroenterology: The Gut Feeling

~With Dr Vinay Thorat

## Introduction

There are endless quips and quotes that tell us that our stomach is not just an organ for digestion. 'You are what you eat'; 'garbage in, garbage out'; 'The way to a man's heart is through his stomach'; 'Gut feeling'; 'Gut instinct'. These are just a few of the many quotes out there. There is more than a grain of truth in these folk aphorisms.

We have come a long way from our looking at the gut only as a food pipe. Food is an important function, of course with the brain controlling what we eat and how we digest it, while the gut informs the brain about hunger and satiety. But their relation goes much beyond food and digestion with an extensive flow of information back and forth between them. The gut nervous system is rightly called the second brain and we shall see how the gut very commonly suffers from *nervous disorders of this second brain*. The gut also plays a major role in emotions and a type of subconscious thinking, what we call instinct. Similarly, mood can decide what we feel like eating and what we eat can affect our state of mind. Intriguingly we have recently started paying attention to the billions of bacteria in our gut, which also seem to talk to our brain.

## The initial simplistic view of the gut and its nervous system

The gastrointestinal system, or the 'gut' in short, is essentially a tube starting from the mouth, going past the food pipe and the stomach, past the small and large bowel to the rectum. Once food enters the tube, various digestive juices are poured in, and the food is churned and propelled along by movements of the gut called peristalsis. All these processes are coordinated by a set of neurons and nerves called the enteric nervous system. The brain controls the gut mainly via the parasympathetic system, which promotes rest, digestion, and growth. When the sympathetic system kicks in, it stops gut activity to allow all resources to be utilized for the *fight or flight* response.

## The present view of the gut and its nervous system

We now know that the gut is much more than a digestive tube, and the enteric nervous system is much more than a local set of nerves to control this digestive tube. There is a complex three-way interaction between the brain, the gut, and the gut microbiome, each affecting the other.

We are aware of how sudden stress or anxiety, sleep and our mood can affect our bowel movements and our digestion. There is now increasing evidence of the gut influencing the brain, directly and indirectly.

The enteric nervous system has almost 500 million cells, more than those in the spinal cord or the peripheral nervous system. Unlike any other organ, this nervous system can work independently of the brain. It is possible that digestion and excretion, being critical for health and survival, got delegated to an independent local manager, rather than constantly have the brain to look at it.

We now have reason to believe that this this huge network of nerves in the gut helps the brain in other activities also, apart from digestion. Most of the messages go from the gut to the brain and not from brain to the gut. Of these, only a small fraction reaches our conscious awareness, like hunger or nausea with poisonous food. Most of the communication is below the radar of consciousness; we are not aware of it.

Scientists now consider this *second brain* as very different. A great deal of our brain's work is at the conscious level; thinking, planning, contemplating, writing, solving puzzles; it is essentially a *thinking brain*. The gut-brain, on the other hand, is mainly a *feeling brain* and works at an unconscious level. It monitors our internal environment; sends information to the brain, affecting memory, emotions, moods, and even motivates us to take certain actions. The gut probably feels or at least influences our emotions. We all know the tight feeling in our stomach when we experience fear or the sensation of 'butterflies' or a 'hollow' in the stomach with anxiety or stress. After all the first emotions of an infant are related to the gut; like the discomfort of hunger and the pleasure of a full stomach. Possibly the gut later evolved to help sense other emotions as well.

The gut may play a very important role in intuitive decision making; it may quickly evaluate the situation in its way and instantaneously tell us the gut feeling. This may confirm or negate the assessment of our thinking brain and guide us away from or towards certain actions or decisions. In some persons, the logical brain is better developed and in some the gut feeling or intuition is more developed. Some people can learn to use them together to great advantage. This strategy of using intuition in conjunction with logical thinking, can be very beneficial, particularly with high-risk decisions.

Scientists believe that our subconscious mind stores data from the past. Some of it is based on our own experiences while some of it is collected from the forms of art we are exposed to, other people's experiences, social media, print media, etc. When faced with a situation that needs instant evaluation, the gut makes use of all this subconscious data and makes it available to the conscious mind through various physiological changes. What we call hunches are probably physical signals from our body, like tenseness in our muscles or a feeling in the gut. These are very rapid assessments of the situation probably using subconscious memories of what we felt in similar situations in the past. Thus 'gut feelings' are a sum of internal sensations, including body temperature, heart rate, muscle tension, and gut sensations.

The enteric nervous system has many similarities with our brain; both having evolved from the same precursor cells; so, they share many of the same chemical messengers or neurotransmitters. Many brain diseases like Parkinson's disease and Alzheimer have their counterpart in the gut; in fact, Parkinson's disease may begin in the gut and gradually spread to the brain. Drugs given for the brain can affect the gut and vice versa. In fact, many of the drugs used for nervous disorders of the brain work for the *nervous disorders of the gut.*

## Gut microbiome

In recent years, a new dimension has been added to the brain-gut connection: the gut microbiome, with the brain, the gut and the gut microbiome, each being able to affect the other. The colony of gut germs or microbiome is like a whole new world within us; it is like a symbiotic partner, joining soon after birth and living with us till we die. It consists of trillions of bacteria, even outnumbering the cells in our body.

The microbiome can be beneficial or harmful, depending or whether the bacteria are pathogenic or helpful ones. The beneficial microbiome protects us against harmful germs, by crowding them out or repelling them and also help in the digestion of food. The gut microbiome has now been linked to various disorders, including inflammatory bowel disease, obesity, diabetes, cardiac disorders, Alzheimer's disease, arthritis, and autoimmune disorders, psychiatric disorders, and autism to name a few.

Various factors have been shown to affect the gut microbiome, including how birth happened, by Cesarian section or normal delivery, whether we were breast-fed or bottle-fed, stress, diet, drugs and antibiotics, geography and, of course, life cycle stages.

The interaction between the gut microbiome and the brain is of relevance. Stress, sleep, mood can all affect the gut microbiome. Just a few hours of stress can instantly change the gut microbiome.

Strangely enough, gut organisms can influence our brain. They can produce many brain neurotransmitters and might be able to influence our moods, our emotions, and our behavior. Serotonin is a good example. This neurotransmitter has a potent effect on our mood, appetite, pain, and sleep and many anti-depressants work by increasing serotonin levels in our brain. It is intriguing, that more than 90 percent of the serotonin in our body is produced by gut bacteria. Studies have shown different effects of bacteria on mood, and now we talk about *psychobiotics* or bacteria which can have a positive influence on mental health.

The gut bacteria may even be able to influence our cravings, i.e. what and how much we eat. It is uncanny, almost as if they are placing an order for what food they want. Imagine, the next time you crave for chocolate, it might be the demand from your gut bacteria!

## Functional gastrointestinal disorders (FGID)

These are the most common group of disorders in gastroenterology. Like any other psychosomatic disorder, function is impaired without any structural or chemical defect. The essential problem is either in the enteric nervous system or in its control by the brain. There are over 30 such disorders, affecting different parts of the gut right from the food pipe to the rectum and anus. They may begin at any age, even infancy, and can change with time.

They are diagnosed by the symptoms; abnormal function of the gut, reduced or excessive motility or secretions and excessive sensitivity or pain. Symptoms range from nausea, vomiting, and belching, to pain, bloating, constipation, and diarrhea, or difficult passage of food or feces.

Like with the other functional disorders, some doctors still consider these as psychological disorders; are uneasy making the diagnosis; may either investigate excessively or may treat the patient dismissively. Being influenced by Descartes' separation of mind from body, they may consider as disease only what they can see, although they do recognize the role of the mind in gut illnesses.

The biopsychosocial model has been proven to be extremely effective in understanding and treating the FGIDs. The biological defect is an abnormal gut physiology, possibly due to genetic predisposition or due to early life events. This interacts with various psycho-social factors and causes symptoms from time to time. Genetic predisposition and early life events can be responsible not just for susceptibility to gut dysfunction. But can also shape psycho-social development, like susceptibility to stress and coping skills.

In many ways, one can consider the FGIDs as mood or anxiety disorders of the second brain, and sure enough, drugs used to treat mood and anxiety disorders of the mind are increasingly being used with excellent results for treatment of these gastrointestinal disorders, including anti-depressants, anti-anxiety, and anti-psychotic medications. Various psychological therapies have been proven very beneficial in the management of FGIDs.

## Nutritional psychiatry

The ancient science of Ayurveda has always laid emphasis on the strong influence of food and digestion on the overall health of the person, including the emotional wellbeing. Ayurveda has pointers on how the choice of food can affect the mood, how certain foods benefit certain personalities, and how the state of the mind in turn can affect your digestion.

We have known for a long time how chocolate can perk up our mood, but in the last few years, modern medicine has started to recognize correlation between mood, emotional wellbeing, and various other foods. Food may have their effect on the brain and mind directly or by modifying the gut flora. The new field of nutritional psychiatry is studying the use food in psychiatric disorders as treatment.

Thus, we have come a long way in understanding the relation of the brain to the 'second brain' in the gut, how they share a common ancestor, are cousins and partners in many ways, and affect each other. We also now recognize the silent partners in our gut, the trillions of germs, who live with us through our whole life, possibly also making some of our decisions for us and for themselves!

## Case 1

We share a case by Dr Vinay Thorat that highlights the predicament of a clinician when the symptoms present as psychosomatic ones, but the puzzle reveals something quite unexpected. The other side of the psychosomatic chasm, in a way.

History taking, as taught in medical colleges, is not even half as complicated as it is in clinical practice. A multitude of nuances come into play when a doctor asks questions that are personal to a patient. I have always been very careful to frame my questions in a way that the cultural and social sensitivities of my patients are not hurt. This turned counterproductive in one case and got permanently etched in my memory.

I was nearing the end of two decades of practice in gastroenterology when a particular gentleman left me scratching my head. He was a 46-year-old priest from a town near Pune and had come to seek an opinion for nagging constipation. No matter what he tried, his constipation always came back. He had tried numerous laxatives and endured various tests, and always came back in time for follow up visits. He had a strange calmness about him and was always very serene in answering all my questions. He had seen other GI specialists before me and was extremely patient throughout.

Celibacy is a part of life for *sadhus* or priests in India and I wondered if that was causing him stress and contributing to his constipation. He was open-minded when I prodded the subject of the mind in his symptoms and tried to explain how his situation might be psychosomatic. He agreed to visit a psychiatrist and was told he had depression and was asked to continue the anti-depressants I had recently started him on. He didn't go back to the psychiatrist but did continue to see me for his quarterly checkups. He would travel a rather formidable distance for each visit, and I always felt a pang of guilt when I sent him away on the antidepressants and laxative without being sure of any diagnosis.

A few months after the gentle priest had seen me, I was having an early dinner with some friends and we were reminiscing about a long past trip we had all taken to a holy town of Bhimashankar. My friend reminded me of the *Gav-jewan* (a sort of free meal served at holy places, for whoever wishes to eat) which we had wolfed down, being totally famished that afternoon. Before we could snap out of the flavours of that afternoon, another friend chuckled, "Hey, and do you remember that filmy looking baba? The one who was passing those little *potlis (pouch bag)* to the others? Discreet, and yet, in the open!" "Oh yes!" I did remember! "I am still wondering what was in those little *potlis*." My friend dramatically rolled his eyes at me before enlightening me with: "Vinay, it was *ganja*. Many of them smoke it..." They were, of course, right. The temple of Lord Shiva in Bhimashankar was a place pulsating with energy. Many devotees of Lord Shiva believe that *ganja* was the preferred smoke of the Lord too. I got lost in a reverie for a few moments, as I remembered my trip to the temple, when suddenly, it struck me! The constipated priest! He prayed at the Shiva temple in his town. Could this finally be the missing piece of the puzzle! I was quite convinced it had to be. I was so excited, I could hardly wait to see him and find out. His appointment was not coming up for a few weeks though. I waited patiently, knowing he would turn up punctually. One bright Wednesday morning, as I walked into my clinic, I saw him outside, patiently waiting to be seen. I planned to broach the topic discreetly as I ushered in the baba and his disciple, because the use of recreational drugs is not uncommon among *sadhus*, but still the topic is a taboo. I could not restrain my eagerness to know though, and the words burst out of my mouth "Does *babaji* smoke *ganja*?" "Yes, of course," replied the disciple nonchalantly. I felt triumphant, as finally I had the answer to the conundrum, which had me perplexed for months. Smoking ganja was the cause of his unremitting constipation. There was no depression. In fact, my antidepressant possibly might have worsened the constipation.

Thankfully, he understood the situation, stopped smoking gradually, his constipation eased away and he soon became symptom-free with a healthy gut and off all medicines.

## Case 2

This is a case from Dr Kinjal Goyal, from the other end of the spectrum. A 39-year-old businessman from New Delhi sought psychotherapy at the behest of his gastroenterologist. He had been suffering from IBS for three years and his flare-ups and episodes were more frequent now, in the last six months, despite compliance with his medicines and following the recommended diet. The tests ordered by the doctors had all confirmed that nothing sinister had been missed.

At the first of the session, he came armed with boxes of papers; simple files were insufficient as he never threw any papers away. After a detailed discussion about the medical aspect of the disease, he commented that his life was perfect in every aspect, except for this one, and he really wanted to get over it. He had a pleasant demeanor and spoke with confidence. His body language revealed something else though. He was fidgety and broke eye contact quickly. His posture was uptight and guarded.

I used the biopsychosocial model for him and explained to him how psychosocial factors might be interacting at this point to worsen his symptoms. With the consent of the patient, the treating doctor was updated after each session and he, in turn, informed me about any change in prescription. Over a few sessions, the patient was asked to draw a timeline of important life changes in the last few years. As he started exploring his personal life more comfortably during therapy, he revealed that he was involved in an extramarital affair. This affair had started three years ago. (The first overlap: The symptoms of IBS had been seen three years ago). It was also revealed later that his wife had found out about the affair around six to seven months ago. (The second overlap: the symptoms had worsened around that time). He had a young child and was distraught with the choices that lay ahead of him.

As the time when awareness of his physical symptoms overlapping with his domestic turbulence came about, CBT was introduced. Through various biofeedback and relaxation techniques, the patient was taught to recognize extreme anxiety and panic triggers and to mitigate them. The patient also undertook marriage counselling along with his wife to find a way ahead. As things started clearing up on the domestic front, his IBS settled substantially. Although he would still have an occasional flare-up, he reported a reduction in the frequency and severity of symptoms by almost 80% (patient's self-report). The patient was relatively symptom-free on a six month follow up.

This case highlights the strong connection between the mind and FGIDs. A treatment plan that included both medical intervention as well as psychotherapy took the patient towards better symptomatic control and disease management.

## Conclusion

The gut is a brain in itself and along with the gut bacteria, has a complex and fascinating interaction with the brain, each influencing the other in ways that are gradually being understood. Treating the Functional Gastrointestinal Disorders as nervous disorders of this brain is helping greatly in understanding and treating these extremely common maladies of mankind.

# Chapter 5

# Endocrinology: Don't Shoot the Messenger

~With Dr Uday Phadke

## Introduction

We like to believe that our thoughts, feelings, and actions are controlled by our thinking logical brain. In fact, though, a tiny part of the brain called the hypothalamus, influences much of our emotions and behavior. It does this by coordinating the two main control systems in our body, the nervous system and the endocrine system. The endocrine system is an ancient system, which uses powerful chemicals called hormones to influence normal bodily functions and all cells, from birth till death. Disorders of the endocrine system are among the leading medical causes of psychiatric illness.

## The hypothalamus and hormones

The nervous system delegates responsibilities to various subdivisions. The enteric nervous system manages feeding and some types of unconscious thinking. Similarly, automatic functions like heart rate, breathing and digestion are managed by the autonomic nervous system, an independent and largely unconscious part of the nervous system. It has two divisions, the sympathetic system for the fight or flight responses and the parasympathetic system for rest, digest and growth. It also controls the body temperature.

The hypothalamus is a part of the primitive brain, which evolved millions of years ago in our worm ancestors. It controls various basic behaviors, like feeding, fighting, fleeing, and reproduction. The size of just an almond, it has clumps of neurons called nuclei, handling different activities. The main functions of the hypothalamus have to do with the autonomic nervous system; the endocrine system and the limbic system maintains our internal environment in the appropriate range needed for health and survival.

We have already had a look at the autonomic nervous system. The second main function has to do with its role as the master gland or the conductor of the endocrine orchestra. Not only does it secrete its own hormones, but it also controls various other hormones, like growth hormone, thyroid, adrenaline, corticotrophin, antidiuretic hormone for water balance, reproductive hormones, oxytocin or the bonding hormone, and melatonin for sleep.

Finally, the hypothalamus functions as a part of the limbic system, which is involved with emotions, sexual behavior, feeding and memory and circuits which deliver a reward for desirable behavior or punishment for undesirable ones.

The hypothalamus is the CEO or the crucial link between the two communication and control systems, the nervous system and the endocrine system, allowing them to work independently or in tandem with one other.

Homeostasis or the processes which keep our internal environment or milieu interior intact is crucial for survival. The body temperature cannot be too high, nor can it be too low. It must be just right, in a narrow range. This holds true for hundreds of other parameters like blood oxygen, glucose, sodium, potassium, blood pressure, and others. The hypothalamus developed in worms to maintain homeostasis. Some experts even feel that the brain evolved to basically remember, predict and plan better and help the hypothalamus manage homeostasis more efficiently or what is called allostasis.

## The two systems for control and communication

Let us take a closer look at our two communication and control systems. The nervous system communicates by electrical messages and neurotransmitters, while the endocrine system sends chemical messages or hormones.

Both neurotransmitters and hormones are chemical messengers controlling and coordinating various body processes and organs. They respond to internal as well as external signals and have a say in almost everything going on in the body, right from our thoughts and feelings, our ability to learn and concentrate, and even our motivations or actions. They sometimes augment each other, sometimes work independently and can influence each other.

There exist feedback loops, which are the basis of many homoeostatic processes. The brain affects the hypothalamus directly or indirectly; the hypothalamus affects the pituitary gland, the pituitary gland affects various hormones, and finally the hormones, tell the brain what they are doing, or the organs on which the hormones are acting, tell the brain. This completes the feedback loop.

The endocrine glands themselves are located all over the body, like the thyroid gland in the neck, the pancreas or the adrenal glands in the abdomen, and the pituitary and hypothalamus in the brain. The two systems are very different in their approach to control. The nervous system is a fast, short-lasting, electrical, focused, and narrow system, while the endocrine is a slow, prolonged, chemical, diffuse, and broad system. They also differ in the actions they control. Neurotransmitters affect voluntary actions (bathing, walking, speaking) as well as involuntary actions (blinking, breathing) but hormones work only on involuntary actions.

The nervous system works like a fast point to point messaging service like a phone call from one person to another or a conference call. The nervous system can send messages only via the nerve to whatever target neuron or muscle or tissue it is connected to and the effect goes away within a fraction of a second.

Hormones act like a broadcasting system to multiple recipients, as the hormones are carried all over the body slowly through the bloodstream. Hormones can affect either specific cells or cells spread out in the body, but the target cells need to have receptors for that hormone. Hormones can inform the brain because it has receptors for many hormones. Hormones can have an effect on multiple organs and sites at the same time; for example, the adrenaline can prepare us to fight or run away by making the heart beat faster and stronger, divert blood supply to muscles and away from non-essential organs like the skin and gut. Similarly, sex hormones can affect various parts and organs of the body simultaneously. The effect of hormones builds up slowly and may last hours or even days.

Let us briefly see the effect of various hormones on the brain, emotions and mind.

## *Thyroid hormone*

Thyroid disorders can clearly affect the brain and the mind in a major way.

Low thyroid can cause excessive sleepiness, impairment of cognition, and slowing of all mental functions including speech. In fact, when an older person comes with brain failure or dementia, one of the treatable causes to be looked for is thyroid deficiency. Some persons can present with depression or even frank psychosis; what used to be called *myxedema madness*.

Thyroid hormone is essential for the development of a baby's nervous system; if there is a deficiency from birth, brain growth is stunted, like a mentally retarded baby. Again, this is so important that now all babies undergo a thyroid check-up at birth to not miss this important preventable cause of mental sub-normality.

Excess thyroxine has effects quite like excessive sympathetic nervous system activation. So, the person may become anxious or nervous, be unable to sleep or get unexplained and severe mood swings, may be irritable and edgy, and even have a frank psychosis. A person with new onset anxiety neurosis should be tested for excess thyroid hormone. They may not be able to concentrate. They tend to be fidgety and hyperactive.

## *Cortisol*

This is the stress hormone and it has many effects on the brain. Low cortisol is known to cause impaired memory, listlessness, fatigue, depression, and psychosis. High cortisol can cause psychiatric abnormalities with irritability, agitation, depression, paranoid psychosis, inability to sleep, and impaired memory and thinking ability. Both steroids and adrenaline have a huge impact on our memory and may explain the effects of acute and chronic stress on memory.

## *Adrenaline*

Excessive adrenaline can cause bouts of palpitations, sweating, headaches, and anxiety with high blood pressure readings – mimicking a panic attack. Low adrenaline may be associated with reduced sex drive and low blood pressure.

## Testosterone

Low testosterone is associated with reduced sexual drive and desire, while high testosterone is associated with aggressiveness. Athletes have been known to have abnormal aggressive behavior and even frank psychosis when they dope themselves with androgenic steroids. When they suddenly stop taking them, they can go into a depression.

## Diabetes

The person with diabetes gets worries, concerns, and fears, right from the time of diagnosis and later as complications threaten. It is a demanding chronic disease and there are legitimate concerns about management, complications, and potential loss of functioning. There is increased incidence of anxiety as well as frank depression in diabetes, both type I or insulin dependent diabetes sometimes seen from childhood, as well as the later onset type II diabetes.

Up to 30–40% diabetics are known to suffer from depression; this was hitherto believed only to occur due to the difficulties encountered in coping with a chronic illness. It's now clear that uncontrolled sugars can itself cause depression and cognitive impairment mimicking dementia. Depression itself can worsen diabetes primarily by changing the stress hormones and the neurotransmitter secretion in the brain. Feeding patterns are also altered and the subsequent weight gain could worsen insulin resistance and diabetes.

The good news is that having good control over sugar levels can help in managing depression, and good control over depression will improve diabetes as well.

One must remain aware that diabetics, on treatment, could suffer from repeated episodes of hypoglycemia (low blood sugar levels). Long duration of diabetes may result in patients not recognizing the usual symptoms (tremors, sweating, hunger) and the patient may instead present as dull and cognitively altered.

Diabetes and obesity often coexist, and both predispose the patient to developing abnormalities of sleep and breathing – obstructive sleep apnea syndrome. There is a disturbed sleep rhythm and intermittent and repeated interruption of oxygen supply to the brain. Diabetes status worsens and the patients often appear inattentive and sleepy through the day as they are catching up on the sleep deficit that they incurred at night.

The presence of this diabetes distress, anxiety and depression can all affect how the patient views treatment and also his compliance towards it.

## Summary

The endocrine system is a versatile and powerful controller of many important involuntary functions in our body. The endocrine and the nervous system often augment and influence each other. The endocrine system is affected by brain activity and psychological factors, and, in turn, can affect brain activity, including thoughts, feelings, behavior, motivation, and many of our unconscious drives. It has an important role to play both in having a healthy mind as well as in many psychiatric disorders.

The endocrine system presents various challenges. Diabetes, although very common and extremely rampant, is still a very challenging disease for a doctor to manage due to various reasons.

## Case 1

Here, we highlight a case by Dr Uday Phadke, a scenario that most endocrinologists must face on a regular basis.

It doesn't take much to sow the seed of distrust or disappointment in the mind of a patient who is facing a chronic ailment which needs a lifetime of monitoring, medication, and self-management: Diabetes Mellitus. Promises of a reversal of diabetes are rife on social media. Nutritionists, quacks, and people who have 'invented' new machines for diabetes reversal don't need to spend too much energy convincing clients to believe them when they say that they hold a cure for the dreaded disease. The patient has just heard from the endocrinologist that diabetes is hard to reverse, and the best way forward is a disciplined lifestyle, measured intake of sugar and carbohydrates, and an exercise regime. The shortcut is naturally more 'tempting'.

I see scores of patients every day, looking for new technology to fix their diabetes. They are willing to spend more money on a short-term treatment plan than accept that simple lifestyle changes and drugs can help them in leading a fulfilling life without any major hindrances.

A 57-year-old businessman had been messaging me every 2–3 minutes from the waiting room. He had missed his appointment which was at 11 am and having walked in at 12 noon, he wanted to be seen immediately. His wife tried to reason with him and kept asking him to drink some water or have a little fruit from the fancy ice box she had in her purse. He would take a bite and wave her off, answering his incessantly beeping phone. In between calls, he would send me a 'gentle' reminder that he was waiting to be seen. Most of my cabins have glass walls and I could glimpse his behavior, in between the other patients that I was seeing.

"Good afternoon doctor!" he greeted me as soon as he entered my cabin. "Good afternoon," I politely replied. He seemed to have an air of having forgiven me for having kept him waiting for 15 minutes, despite him having missed his appointment by more than an hour. I glanced at his latest reports and noticed a rise in blood sugar levels, both fasting and postprandial. His HbA1C had risen too. On asking him why the sudden increase, he said he had stopped his medicines recently. He was now on a specialized diet that could reverse diabetes and was also using a contraption that needed to be worn for a particular time in the day to help with blood sugar levels. The increase in sugar levels was temporary, he told me. It would be perfectly in control next time. His wife noticed my incredulous expression and silently urged me to change her husband's mind. I warned him about the dangers of stopping his medicines so abruptly and told him that he could try the new diet plan while taking the medicines. We could review the blood sugar levels frequently and reduce the dose gradually if the diet did help. I also offered to send him authentic data about the machine he was using, as contrary to the manufacturer's claims, it had absolutely no effect on diabetes. Everything fell on deaf ears. He didn't budge. Eventually, I wrote out a new prescription and implored him to reconsider taking the medicines. As they walked out, his wife asked him if they could at least buy the medicines. "Oh please. Don't fall for all this marketing gimmick. It's just a way for them to keep earning money. Nowadays doctors simply don't want you to get off medicines. How will they get their cuts from pharma companies otherwise? I know what I am doing. It will work, just wait and watch."

I inadvertently, heard this exchange and felt a heaviness creep over me. I knew I had done nothing wrong, but some patients make you feel hopeless and helpless. I took a deep breath, put on my best smile for the next patient, and went on with my day.

It took three weeks for the call to come. The same gentleman had been admitted to the ICU with very high blood sugar levels and hypertension. It took us a couple of days to bring down the sugar and blood pressure. He was shifted out to a room. I saw him that evening on my rounds. I almost felt like saying 'I told you so', but medical ethics has taught me to remain calm, composed, and provide the best treatment that I could.

I expected some remorse from the patient for having gone against medical advice. Instead, with tears glimmering in his eyes, he said to me "I don't know what I have done to deserve this, doctor". I followed the diet, did everything advised to beat this damned disease, and yet, I failed. I am so tired now. I just feel like giving it all up. How much longer can I fight it ?"

My anger gave way to pity. Here was a man who had the resources and wherewithal to buy the best medicines for a lifetime. He had a wife who cared. He had everything, except faith in medicine. A deluge of social media posts, misleading promises, and 'quick fixes' led him to believe that he was being smart and taking care of himself by avoiding medicines and following the miracle diet. He had invested all his emotional and physical energy in a direction that led him to a 'dead' end, although not literally, thank God! Now, he felt that no matter what he did, diabetes was not in his control. He felt dwarfed by the disease. He felt let down. Although he had been told that this method will hurt him in the long run, he found it even harder to trust me now. It wasn't about me. It was about his inability to trust again.

Irrational beliefs can really be detrimental to the patient. This person had ideas of grandiosity and held a strong irrational belief that no matter what doctors said, he could, and he should be able to conquer his disease. This false belief made him think that lifelong medication and monitoring blood sugar levels was undesirable and unnecessary. When a patient doesn't accept that he needs treatment, he fights it with all that he has. When that fails, it saps him of his energy and leaves him feeling low, even depressed.

Diabetes, like almost every other disease, has varying levels of severity. A diet may help someone who is, maybe pre-diabetic and harm someone who has had the disease for many years and suddenly stops his medicines. One solution doesn't fit everyone. Going against medical advice is risky for everyone though. Not only does it harm the body, but it also unsettles the patient's mind. Reduced compliance towards the prescribed treatment leads to more complications in the long run.

This is where trust plays a major role. Being able to trust a doctor is paramount in the treatment of any chronic illness. This partnership between doctor and patient leads to the best long-term care.

## Case 2

This case highlights how disturbances in the endocrine system can lead to various symptoms that lead a patient to specialists in different fields.

Mrs N was a 26 year old lady, a doctor, who had surgery to remove her thyroid glands for a thyroid cancer. and had recovered well post-surgery. She was placed on a relatively high dose of thyroxine as per guidelines after such surgery. Both parents were senior doctors.

She got married and her husband was studying for his super specialization in another city. Soon after her baby was born, Mrs N started getting multiple physical symptoms, including fluctuations in heart rate, dizziness and painful and heavy menstruation. The patient's father, a senior pediatrician, was convinced that the high dose of thyroxine was causing the symptoms and they were, of course, described in persons with excess thyroid hormone. The endocrinologist assured them that it was unlikely to be due to the thyroxine, as she had tolerated that dose for years and that it was imperative, she continue the high dose to prevent a cancer from recurring.

So she and her family looked elsewhere for the cause of the distressing symptoms. They consulted a cardiologist first. The variation in heart rate was studied with an objective outlook but was found to be of non-cardiac origin. Long term Holter studies were conducted, but they revealed nothing. The patient ended up getting hospitalized, five times for various symptoms; each time without any explanation or relief. They googled and did find some mention of similar symptoms with prolonged high dose of thyroxine.

As she later started getting bouts of dizziness, they consulted a neurologist next. The neurologist examined and investigated her and opined that the dizziness was not due to any ear problem or organic brain disorder and was likely a form of migraine, aggravated by possible stress after the baby was born. This explanation was not acceptable to her parents though and seeing their daughter so unwell, they got more and more involved. They started scouting the internet, in the hope of finding an explanation for her symptoms. They sought opinions from doctors in other cities too, all the while hoping to find the elusive answer.

Eventually, the endocrinologist also spoke to them about seeing a mental health therapist and exploring the possibility of a role of the mind in her suffering. This is where things changed, although still not as dramatically as one might expect. The parents, coming from strong medical backgrounds, had strong inhibitions about what they considered 'banishing' their daughter to the dungeons of the mind. They believed being a clear-headed and intelligent person, their daughter could not get mental health issues. After all other doors got closed, they reluctantly met a therapist and started psychotherapy.

Note the use of the word, 'they' in this case. More than the patient, the parents needed to undergo basic psychoeducation. Once they understood that psychosomatic does not mean 'fake', they were more amenable to the treatment and allowed their daughter to undergo this therapy, which they had not understood in the past.

As therapy progressed, various issues came to light. The patient was intelligent and used to being independent. Marriage, motherhood, surgery, and dependence on medication had slowly taken away her sense of control. Although she felt helpless in the wake of things, she tried desperately not to give up control. As an anesthesiologist, she understood her symptoms well and read deeply into them each time any symptom surfaced. Her anxiety stemmed from knowing exactly what all could go wrong. She admitted to having made a pouch of emergency medicines for bradycardia (low heart rate), tachycardia (high heart rate), dizziness, headaches, menorrhagia (excessive bleeding during her periods), and a few other pills. She would carry this pouch everywhere with her, even within the house. What started off as a precautionary measure, had slowly taken over her mind.

Having been to various doctors and having seen her own reports come back near normal, she needed to believe her symptoms were real; she needed to feel validated from someone else apart from her parents, who of course believed in her suffering. She had started feeling like an imposter without even realizing it.

Therapy helped her come face to face with her symptoms, her personality, the void in her personal life, and helped her regain her lost confidence. Multiple hospital admissions had left her feeling scared and helpless. Eventually, the patient learnt to distribute her symptoms along the disease—illness axis and learnt to trust her treating doctor more. The parents backed off and gave her the space she needed to take care of herself. With renewed confidence and restructuring of her thoughts and behavior, she soon had an almost complete remission of her symptoms. She got off the extra medicines and became more compliant with the medicines that she needed to be on. She did have a relapse six months down the line but got relief again with psychotherapy.

This is just one of the multitude of cases that the field of endocrinology presents. The hormones that rule our body also have a major voice in our heads. In the second case therapy could succeed, because the patient was not asked to choose one from psychotherapy and medical treatment. The therapist and the medical professionals worked hand in hand; one helping her achieve the maximum possible level of emotional wellbeing, and the other keeping her health optimum with the appropriate medicines.

# Chapter 6
# Cardiology: Straight from the Heart

~With Dr Yash Lokhandwala
and Dr Aniruddha Vyas

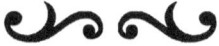

Although psychology and medicine have various crossovers in multiple fields, almost all, if one may take the larger picture, nowhere else is the mind-body connect as visible as in the field of cardiology. Fear, anger, grief, stress, and sadness have been associated with cardio-pulmonary symptoms since ancient times. People thus believed, since ancient times, that the heart was the seat of all emotions. A lexicon of metaphors has been in use since ancient times, which are still in use today; 'heartache' and 'heartbreak' being the most used ones. Generosity is defined as people being 'large-hearted' while empathy is often described as 'my heart went out to...' The heart and its association with emotions is truly a thing of legend. Songs have been sung and ballads written, endless movies have been made using 'heart' in the name itself. We have all seen movies in which an intense outburst of anger triggers a massive heart attack. And there are scores of movies, in which, after the person suffers a heart attack, the treating doctor tells the relatives, with a grave expression, "He needs to be kept away from any kind of stress".

The brain seems to be the only organ capable of rational thinking and so emotional matters are attributed to the heart, particularly since everyone has experienced how the heart reacts to various emotional disturbances. Feeling the heart racing when excited or scared, skipping a beat when startled, and experiencing chest pain when stressed, have all forged this connection of the emotions with the heart. In general, people make a distinction between a logical person, who thinks and makes decisions with his brain and an emotional person, who decides with his heart.

Another aspect of cardiac psychology is the distress a person feels after getting diagnosed with a cardiac ailment. Sudden, unexpected cardiac events like a heart attack or cardiac arrest can lead to extreme anxiety, fear of death, and sometimes post-traumatic stress disorder too. What is interesting to note is that even after the cardiac ailment is cured, the anxiety may linger, sometimes below the surface. Patients with chronic cardiac ailments also have long-term psychological issues. There is some evidence to link certain behavioral patterns and personality traits with a higher risk of ischemic heart disease.

The first step for a cardiologist is to understand if the patient's symptoms are due to organic heart disease or psychological. Making a mistake could be disastrous or end up in unnecessary anxiety and investigations and expenses. A person coming with chest pain and difficulty in breathing could be having a heart attack or a panic attack and the two conditions need a very different line of management.

It is important to keep in mind the possibility of heart disease and psychological issues coexisting; each affecting the other. We need to look for and address psychological issues in persons with heart disorders to improve the overall wellbeing of the patient. Getting a heart attack or a diagnosis of a serious heart ailment or suddenly getting a burst of palpitations or missing a few beats can lead to intense anxiety and fear. A patient who suffers a sudden cardiac event and is hospitalized, even briefly, may experience post-traumatic stress disorder. The combination of a near-fatal experience, losing one's sense of control, the financial burden, all affect the patient's wellbeing long after the disease has been stabilized medically. On the other hand, stress can clearly aggravate or even trigger cardiac problems, like angina or a heart attack, and rhythm disorders. In addition, psychological factors can influence compliance and acceptance of treatment.

Sometimes psychological problems can really break one's heart. The *broken heart syndrome* is known to cardiologists as Takotsubo Cardiomyopathy. Intense grief, stress, domestic violence, and severe medical illness or extreme physical stress can make the heart mimic a heart attack, with chest pain and breathlessness and abnormal ECG. The Echocardiogram shows the characteristic ballooning of the heart, so it looks like a takotsubo or 'octopus pot'. An angiogram is needed to show that the arterial supply to the heart is normal, unlike in a heart attack. It is thought that a sudden surge of adrenaline and sympathetic nervous system stimulation stuns the heart muscle and makes it beat abnormally. It is luckily a temporary condition, though it may need treatment by drugs as well as psychotherapy. Peculiarly, it tends to occur mainly in women, more often post-menopausal.

The distinction may not always be easy. For example, in a patient with sudden bursts of abnormal heart beating called arrhythmias, stress can trigger episodes. We, of course, treat both; judicious drugs for the heart rhythm and stress management techniques for the mind, but it can be difficult to decide which one to focus on; the heart rhythm or the stress. Management decisions can be tricky indeed in such patients.

From a psychological perspective, cardiac psychotherapy is a very important segment in psychosomatic medicine. Cognitive behavior therapy, rational emotive behavior therapy, and the use of the biopsychosocial model have proven to be efficacious in helping cardiac patients achieve symptomatic relief and improve compliance with ongoing medical treatment.

Here we discuss two cases shared by Dr Lokhandwala and Dr Vyas, to highlight the importance of the psychological state in heart problems.

## *Case 1*

On a busy Monday, as I rushed up the stairs towards my outpatient clinic on the first floor, wading through the crowd of patients and caregivers, with the constant background hum of a typical Indian hospital, I threw a fleeting glance towards the patients waiting to see me. A tall gentleman with off white shiny hair, over a seasoned forehead skin, smiled at me. He had a soothing and learned look, with his warm looking brown sweater worn over a white shirt and khaki trousers. I smiled back at him and continued my 'science of deduction' as my eyes glided on towards an elderly lady beside him, with similar white hair, but a worried countenance and a wrinkled frown on her forehead. I construed that she was his wife.

I went into my cabin and getting ready to see the first patient, I called out the first name on the list, as I pulled open the door. It was the elderly couple, who stood up and walked in. I said to them "Hello, I hope I didn't make you wait for long." His reply was a nod with a broad smile, revealing his shiny white teeth and broad jawline. As he stood up, I noticed he was agile, well built, at least, half a foot taller than me. I felt he was likely an athlete in the past. He greeted me with a firm handshake and followed a pleasant respecting etiquette as he entered my office.

After exchanging pleasantries, I went through the medical details. He had a PhD, was a retired IIT professor, presently seeing his 95th spring, and had come to seek my opinion on a recent deterioration in his health due to dwindling heart function. I was surprised, as his mental sharpness, his physique and broad chest made him look much younger and unlikely to have significant cardiac issues. In reality, due to a massive heart attack three decades ago, he had a very weak heart, which was able to pump hardly 20 percent of the expected capacity. He also had a rhythm abnormality called permanent atrial fibrillation, with chaotic heart beats. A pacemaker-defibrillator device had been implanted in his chest and the conduction pathway in the heart (AV Node) had been ablated to reduce the racing heart rate. The idea of the pacemaker was to kick in if the heart stopped beating and the defibrillator to shock any chaotic heart beats of ventricular fibrillation. His wife instantly picked up the worry, evident in my eyes. She was aware of his overall health and was anxious about the recent worsening. But the gentleman continued to smile rather confidently. I adjusted some medicines, the least and the most I could do at that point of time with the state of his heart. I tried to think of words to comfort him, but I realized that he needed neither my sympathy nor empathy. He was a tenacious person.

Thankfully, over the next few weeks, with the treatment changes we made, his recent deterioration reversed. Over the next few days and months, I developed a close connection with the couple. They lived not far from my home, in a cozy, old-fashioned bungalow. I learnt that their children were highly educated and were now settled in the USA. I met them frequently at their home. The man had rather astounding achievements in his lifetime. He was a mountaineer and was in the first Indian team expedition to attempt to scale Mount Everest in the 1960s. Using an old projector, he projected slides as he narrated the story of his expedition. I got awestruck when he told me that Tenzing Norgay was amongst his close friends. He did not sound even remotely sad about the fact that despite all their efforts and preparations, the team had failed just short of the summit. As a young man, I was captivated by the way he viewed his life. I realized that failing to reach a particular summit in our own personal expeditions in life should not feel like a failure. The very attempt to venture on an expedition should feel like achieving the summit itself. I learnt from him that one should never stop the ascent in life and call an expedition off and treat each forward step as a milestone. Over the next two years, my relationship with him transformed from a doctor to a friend.

As his health declined further with progressing age, I suggested that his children take the couple to the United States, which they did. After a few months in the USA, more in hospital than at home, he passed away peacefully, wearing his usual smile and surrounded by his children and loving wife. He never lost his mental strength in his lifetime, not even at the time of his demise. As a cardiologist, I deal with patients suffering from heart failure all the time. I know how hard it must feel be to be drowning in your own body, as the lungs fill up with fluid.

He never complained about anything, about not being able to reach the Everest summit, about his ailing heart, his ageing body, or about living alone with his wife in India with the children settled abroad. He was content with whatever he did and achieved in his life. I have seen even more accomplished people complaining and feeling sad about their lives. His athletic build and physique helped him, but in the final count, it was his sound mind that gave him the resilience to face the hardships of his life with a smile. Acceptance brought him peace and gave him the strength to live with his extremely weak heart for over three decades, with a smile which even death could not take away.

## Case 2

**Our second case highlights the emotional effects of a malfunctioning implanted device in a patient who was otherwise mentally strong and rather resilient.**

Sometimes, some interventions performed with the intent to make things better can lead to the worsening of a patient's physical and emotional wellbeing. I remember clearly this 78 year old gentleman, full of energy and zeal. He was among the most affluent people in the city, actively involved in his busines. He also had a group of friends with whom he would spend many nights at the club, sharing a drink and friendly banter. He suffered from liver and kidney disease apart from a weak heart, pumping only at one third the expected capacity for his age. I regularly encounter people with weak hearts and rhythm disturbances and find myself drawn into their struggles. Their struggles seem as real to me as if they were mine.

I did not know him for very long. My first encounter with him was rather accidental. His son sought my urgent appointment for an implanted cardioverter-defibrillator, which was apparently giving him unnecessary and inappropriate shocks. The device is implanted to give a shock to and correct the heart, only when it beats chaotically and threatens life. In his case, however, the machine was misfiring and giving shocks every now and then, when not needed, as his heart was beating perfectly normally. These are strong electrical shocks and give a jolt to the heart and the body. As I entered the emergency room, I saw on the bed, a weak, panting, and perspiring man with a receding white hairline. The room was unusually warm, and that, combined with his fear, made him sweat profusely. He cupped his palm just below the left shoulder, as if to implore the implanted device not to fire. He was replying to all my queries peacefully, when suddenly, his face contorted in pain. The machine had fired again.

I suspected the shocks were inappropriate ones and placing a magnet over the skin, I checked what the device was doing. Indeed it was working erratically and giving unnecessary shocks and I switched it off. The device had been implanted three months ago, to prevent serious consequences like brain damage or death if the heart suddenly started beating chaotically. Unfortunately, the electrical wire placed inside the heart had got displaced and was causing frequent, unpredictable and unwarranted shocks, despite the heart beating normally. I told him that the only way out was to operate again and change the electrical wire.

After having gone through the malfunction and the painful shocks, it wasn't an easy decision for him and he and his family sought some more opinions. They finally told me they had decided to get repeat surgery at the hospital where it had been implanted earlier. He called me cheerfully a few days after the repeat surgery. Unfortunately, this happiness was not to last for long.

One Sunday around 5:45 am, I got a phone call and answered automatically with sleepy eyes, without even looking at who it was. The voice sounded familiar but shaky and scared. It was his son again calling to tell me his father had got a shock again. I rushed to the hospital, thinking he must have had a life-threatening rhythm disturbance, making the machine fire and save his life. I checked the machine again with the magnet over the skin and was shocked myself and disappointed to see that even this shock was unwarranted and happened despite the heart beating perfectly well. They could hardly believe me as they had thought the worst was behind them.

I switched off the device again to stop the unwarranted shocks. This time it was another technical glitch. I must mention here that such devices are implanted all over the world and generally work as programmed and probably have saved more human lives than any other single medical invention. This was a freak incident causing him repeated trouble.

He didn't bother to even look at the published evidence and the scientific data I uttered in favour of the device. I gave him the same option as before, expecting him to agree to repeat the surgery, this time under my care. A few months passed but they did not contact me and I thought maybe they had gone elsewhere again to get it done.

One day, I got a call from his son, sounding very dejected. He told me that his father was no longer his usual self; seemed depressed most of the time, had lost weight, had stopped tending to his business affairs and had even stopped meeting his friends in the club. He probably was weighed down by the decision he had to make, neither choice palatable. He could not bear to think of the painful shocks again, but not doing anything meant facing a daily risk of dying suddenly. The common denominator was fear and he had to choose one. He consulted a psychiatrist and took the prescribed medicines to help with his anxiety and insomnia. They did help him to sleep better, but he could not decide and remained depressed.

He finally came over to meet me with his son and nephew. I noticed a dreadful change in the two months since I had seen him. His facial expression was blank, his beard shabby and overgrown, his eyes sunken and lifeless with dark circles. His clothes were untidy and unkempt., a rather striking change from the earlier well-groomed man. After a long silence, he cleared his throat and tried to speak, but was on the verge of tears. I offered him a glass of water and waited. In a few minutes, he regained his composure, looked straight in my eyes and said, "Take out the device. I don't want it." I was taken aback and didn't really know what to say. His son explained that after two months of giving it a thought, he had finally made up his mind to take it out and not implant again.

I started to explain why it might not be a safe option to take the device out, but he interrupted me and in the same calm tone repeated the request, "Can you take out this device?" I sighed, thought a while, looked straight back in his eyes and said, "Yes, I can." His eyes suddenly lit up and the shadow of a smile crept in.

We spent a day in various formalities as we were potentially putting him at risk of sudden death. A detailed informed consent was taken from him, his family, and the hospital superintendent for medico-legal issues. The next day, as I saw him lying on the catheterization table, I was surprised to see how cheerful and chirpy he was during the procedure. As it was done under local anesthesia, he was fully alert and behaving as if a curse was being taken off from him.

Once the device was taken out, I saw pure magic happen. He regained his zeal and enthusiasm and interest in all his earlier activities. He started to wake up early for a cup of morning tea in his large courtyard and then attend to his business affairs and again would end his days at the club with his friends and his trusted glass of Scotch, despite my appeals to protect his liver and heart. We became friends and two years have passed since then without any untoward incident.

For a man who had always held the reins of his life in his own hands, the ICD had taken away all sense of control. The uncertainty and pain of the shocks made him feel miserable and helpless. The first time he had erred on the side of caution and had followed sound medical advice. But when the device failed again, he had to make a hard decision. Neither did he wish to live with undesirable shocks, nor did he want to live under the cloud of the fear of sudden death. The choice was one that he probably never thought he would have to make. A close brush with one's mortality does lead to serious introspection and, in this case, the patient chose to have a life free of painful shocks, even if it meant the risk of a shorter life and sudden death. This decision finally gave him the freedom he was used to. The freedom to choose his life, and, in a manner, his death. The fatal arrhythmia did not happen, but even if it did, he was prepared for it mentally.

As his treating doctors, we knew that the risk he was taking was a big one. But we also realized that the price he would have paid to avoid the risk would be a greater one. He took responsibility for his decision and chose freedom. The strength of the mind shone through yet again, allowing us to take a step back and revel in the many layers that bind the heart and the mind.

The understanding of the overlap between psychology and cardiology has far-reaching effects on the treatment and outcome for patients. Working hand in hand, cardiologists and psychologists can use the biopsychosocial model most effectively and ensure not only compliance but also a better quality of life for the patients.

# CHAPTER 7
# Dizziness: A New Spin

## Introduction

You are crossing a street and turn your head to look to the side and suddenly feel as if someone gave you a big push; or, in the kitchen, you reach up to get a jar from the top shelf and suddenly the room spins violently, and you almost fall. The list is endless, tying your laces, lying down to sleep, or turning in bed in the middle of the night. What if these spins happened only sometimes and unpredictably? What if the doctors seemed unsure of the cause; one calling it blood pressure, another spondylosis, the third blaming blood supply to the brain, and yet another talking vaguely about a fluid problem in the inner ear?

It is not at all surprising that a high number of patients with recurrent vertigo develop anxiety or depression. "Could I fall? What if I were to fall?" Just such thoughts can affect your balance and increase the risk of falling.

Vestibular disorders cause sensations of spinning, dizziness, or imbalance. Vertigo is defined as *a false sensation of movement (often spinning), whereas dizziness best describes a feeling of disorientation in space without the sensation of movement, and unsteadiness is feeling off-balance when standing or walking.* Whilst they are often assumed to be due to ear problems, not infrequently such symptoms are caused by problems affecting the brain, and exacerbated by psychological factors such as anxiety.

The interaction between the mind and vestibular disorders has increasingly been recognized in recent years. Indeed, vestibular disorders often cause anxiety and even depression and various psychological disorders can also affect our balance. Anxiety can itself cause dizziness or feelings of imbalance, even without problems in the ear or brain.

## The *miracle* of standing and walking without falling

We often take for granted how challenging standing upright and walking actually is. Any engineer will tell you that a ground-hugging car is less likely to topple over than a double-decker bus. No one designs a chair with only two legs. Then why did man get himself into this precarious position on two legs?

There are many causes proposed, but the main advantage is that it frees our hands, for example, to use tools, gives us a better view of our surroundings, and allows a more efficient way of moving, namely walking and running.

What do we do about being top-heavy with a narrow base of support and constantly being at risk of losing balance? Like gyroscopes and accelerometers, which tell the pilot when an airplane is turning and tilting, we have a fantastic balance system which constantly checks and corrects our balance and our centre of mass. It is only because the brain constantly assesses and makes adjustments that we maintain our balance on two legs. Every step we take, we actually tend to fall forward; we break the fall with the front foot and get ready for the next step. Learning to balance, stand, walk, run, and hop is no mean achievement, as watching the efforts and time put in by any baby will tell you. Of course, it helps that babies are not deterred by repeated falls. The fear of heights and falls comes only later in life, once the 'stakes' become higher. With their osteoporosis and higher risk of fracture and incapacitation, the elderly are particularly worried about falls.

The brain constantly evaluates the risks and adjusts our posture and gait accordingly. If you have ever stood or seen someone stand at the edge of a cliff or a ledge, you will know how our body and legs become stiff, our steps shorter, and our eyes remain glued to the ground. Anxiety and fear can drastically change our stance and gait, in health as well as in disease. These adaptations are meant to reduce the chances of a fall, but when they become habitual, they can paradoxically increase our risk of falling. The mere thought of what may happen if you fall, can itself lead to a fall.

## How balance and the vestibular system work

Balance depends on multiple streams of information reaching the brain; the eyes informing about how the world looks; straight or tilted or upside down; the sensory system informing us how the body and legs are aligned, and the inner ear informing us about tilting or movement, up, down, front or back, or turning.

Using all this information, the brain makes a 'best guess' as to what is happening and gives us our sense of balance, orientation, direction, and speed of movement. Mistakes can happen when there is a wrong message coming in from the ear, or if the brain interprets the message wrongly.

The common causes of dizziness stemming from the ear are:

- BPPV, due to small calcium particles in the inner ear getting displaced into the wrong place.
- Vestibular Neuritis or labyrinthitis due to infection of the inner ear.
- Meniere's disease, a rare inner ear disorder.

The common causes of dizziness stemming from the brain are:

- Vestibular migraine, a 'dizzy' variant of migraine.
- Stroke, brain tumour, demyelination.

## The holistic approach to anxiety and vestibular disorders

For many years, vestibular disorders were thought to be either due to the ear or the brain. Dizziness without any abnormality found in the ear or brain was often thought to be psychological in origin ('psychogenic'). We now realize how important the mind is in vestibular disorders, both as a cause and a consequence of vestibular symptoms. This tight relationship has an anatomical basis – the regions of the brain areas processing anxiety and vestibular input are closely related to and affect each other. These psychological factors are potentially treatable if recognized early and handled appropriately.

## Why do dizzy patients get anxious or depressed?

There are many reasons why vertigo and dizziness are particularly distressing. For one, they threaten our basic need for independent mobility, lead to a loss of control, and may bring into question the very state of our being.

Vestibular function is our sixth sense, working below the radar, and is often taken for granted. Unlike other sensations like vision and hearing, it is difficult to characterize and describe.

The unpredictability and severity of a vertigo attack or sudden fear of a fall is difficult to handle. Because the cause of the symptoms may not be accessible with a simple test, the doctor's visit commonly ends with the person feeling misunderstood, undervalued, and dismissed. Not knowing clearly what it is, how, when, and if it will go away, can be very disconcerting. 'Googling' for causes when no explanation has been offered by the doctor may further worsen the confusion and anxiety.

Persistent or recurrent dizziness or vertigo can lead to other secondary psychosomatic symptoms like fatigue, tiredness, and even an inability to think clearly. When the vestibular system is functioning normally, the brain does not have to give any thought to balance or orientation; it occurs automatically. But the dizzy or unsteady person has to make conscious efforts to maintain balance and orientation, and may have less energy for other tasks, and so often fatigues quickly.

## Common psychiatric problems in dizzy patients

Panic attacks, anxiety, depression, and a condition called PPPD (Persistent Perceptual-Postural Dizziness) are the main psychological disorders in dizzy patients. Even if there is a known disorder like BPPV or migraine, if symptoms seem to be out of proportion to the nature of the disorder or the person looks emotionally distressed, one needs to assess for co-existing anxiety or depression.

## Psychological issues in the first attack of vertigo

The first attack of vertigo, whatever the cause, can be very scary and distressing, with spinning, dizziness, and imbalance, along with symptoms like nausea, vomiting, and sweating. The abrupt onset of the symptoms, and their severity, may raise a suspicion of a heart attack or stroke, leading to admission to an emergency setting or even an intensive care unit. The more the initial anxiety, the more the chances that the person will keep having symptoms, after months or even years. These residual symptoms are usually due to PPPD rather than persistent vestibular nerve dysfunction.

If one can reassure the patient and minimize anxiety in the acute stage, one can prevent the emergence of chronic vestibular symptoms.

## Psychological issues in repeated attacks of vertigo

The most common causes of repeated attacks of vertigo are disorders like BPPV, vestibular migraine, or Meniere's disease.

A smaller group has an isolated anxiety disorder, particularly panic attacks. After cardiac or pulmonary causes, vestibular problems are the second most common symptom in panic disorder.

Anxiety or depression is seen in over half the cases of migraine or Meniere's. It is comparatively less prevalent in BPPV, where the symptoms are briefer and are triggered by defined head movements, that the patient can predict and learn to avoid. But in migraine or Meniere's, the attacks do not seem under the patient's control and so the anxiety is more.

## Psychological issues in chronic dizziness

Almost one in three chronically dizzy or unsteady patients have psychiatric disorders, especially generalized anxiety or less commonly depression.

Minor abnormalities on vestibular testing or on balance tests need to be interpreted with caution in such patients to avoid incorrect diagnosis or further unnecessary tests.

## PPPD or persistent postural-perceptual dizziness

This is an exceedingly common functional disorder of the balance system. It used to be called subjective dizziness because the patient feels dizzy, but the doctor finds nothing to explain it. It is not a purely psychiatric disorder like anxiety or depression, as there may be a precipitating vestibular disorder, such as BPPV, vestibular neuritis, or even syncope or fainting. An attack of vertigo or fainting often induces transient anxiety, with the person adopting a more cautious gait and becoming more watchful in general of their body and relying more on visual information for balance.

Most people go on to recover after a single or even recurrent episodes of vertigo. Why some persons go on to develop PPPD is not entirely clear. It may be related to the severity of the attack, and the initial level of anxiety and fear. More likely these persons are, by nature, more sensitive, more analytical or inquisitive, and more anxious or introverted. In these persons, the transient protective response persists and become excessive and maladaptive. Their brain misinterprets and creates a false sense of movement or orientation. The situation turns into a vicious circle with worsening imbalance and anxiety and loss of confidence.

The symptoms are persistent and typically last over three months, almost daily with some ups and downs. The patient typically feels non-specifically dizzy or off-balance, and fears he/she may fall, though he/she has no objective signs or obvious loss of balance and does not actually fall. The patient may feel as if he/she is swaying to and fro, like in a boat, even when lying in bed, although these symptoms are typically worse when the patient is standing or walking. The walking may be affected, with slow and cautious steps. The symptoms are often triggered or suddenly worsened by certain movements or postures. They tend to occur in certain provocative situations, for example, large empty rooms, crowded places, or in a mall or a cinema. The person may drive a car normally and suddenly feel dizzy at a traffic signal, when the cars buzz past.

There are often additional cognitive symptoms such as fatigue, impaired concentration, fear of going out alone, and avoidance of places or situations that could trigger or worsen the balance. Such avoidance may be detrimental to recovery, and negatively affect the work and social aspects of their lives. Just as all roads lead to Rome, the initial trigger can be any vestibular disorder and one needs to actively prevent the development of PPPD in all such patients.

## Treatment of PPPD

PPPD can be successfully treated ideally with a multi-pronged approach, even in patients who have had symptoms for a very long time, though not everyone will improve. The chances of improvement are better if the patient understands the mechanisms underpinning their symptoms, feels reassured that the disorder is not life-threatening or progressive and that there are defined treatments for it. In order to fully engage the patient in such understanding, the physician's explanation of the condition must first align with the patient's own interpretation of the disorder, such that a common understanding can be reached.

Various forms of physiotherapy may be effective, in which the patient is encouraged to move in a graded fashion. Often they need psychological support like counselling and CBT, and careful use of drugs like SSRIs or anti-depressants. Many patients can improve and regain their balance and confidence.

### Case 1

A pleasant 52-year-old lawyer came to me last week for loss of confidence in balance and intermittent dizziness. Two years ago, while playing badminton, he bent down to pick up the shuttle and suddenly felt dizzy. He felt a fleeting spin for a few seconds when he lay down in bed and once while rolling over in the bed. His family doctor diagnosed him to have vertigo and prescribed anti-vertigo drugs for a week.

Four months later, he had this transient dizziness once again, and, thereafter, started feeling intermittently as if he was losing balance towards the right side when walking. He would intermittently feel fear and his sleep also got disturbed. He got an MRI of his brain and cervical spine, and MR angiogram to check the blood supply to his brain and showed it to a neurologist, a neurosurgeon, as well as a psychiatrist, but did not feel better.

I saw before me an anxious person, with otherwise no abnormality in his vestibular or neurological examination. His balance seemed perfectly normal. When I was speaking with him, twice he uttered the words *loss of confidence*. The first time he said he had lost confidence in walking but the second time he only said he had lost confidence. Picking up a possible clue, I asked him how this dizziness had affected his day-to-day life as a person or as a lawyer.

Now he opened up and told me quite innocently that because of this lack of confidence he had declined an invitation to become a judge. He said he was not sure, because of this imbalance, whether he would be able to handle his increased responsibilities as a judge.

I wonder whether he probably had an attack of BPPV to begin with and the subsequent worry about being able to cope with increased job responsibility as a judge induced PPPD. I have seen persons having a similar experience after a job promotion or when responsibility increases, often after the sudden demise of a father. Just as doubts about balance can worsen balance, it sometimes happens that feeling a lack of confidence in handling a new responsibility can somehow get transformed into a lack of confidence in balance. I hope that with therapy, we might empower him to take on the job of a judge.

## Case 2

Mrs Bhide was an active 75-year-old; widowed for the past five years. Her children in the USA visited her every year. Every morning she went for a walk in the park and conducted a laughter club. She managed her day-to-day grocery shopping as well as bank activities.

One day, when she woke up and sat up in bed, she was suddenly thrown backwards into her bed. She got very scared and just could not understand what had happened. She lay quietly in bed for a minute and then tried to get up again. Again she was thrown back. Now, she tried to turn onto one side and felt a violent spin, so she just lay still in bed on her back, not daring to make any movement. Without turning her head, she stretched out her hand to the side table and groped for her mobile phone and managed to find it and then called her neighbour. The lady promptly came down and tried to make her sit up but couldn't, and so she called their family doctor, who told them to get her admitted to a nearby big hospital.

She was taken to hospital in an ambulance and wheeled into the casualty section. The duty doctor came, did a brief history and examination, got urgent MRI brain and other tests done, told her that it was probably a stroke, and sent her to the ICU, where she spent the day. She hardly slept at night in the ICU, terrified by the beeping and other noises. The next morning she could get up in bed, though she still felt unsteady and dizzy intermittently.

An orthopaedic consultant felt that the attack was due to cervical spondylosis (wear and tear in her neck spine) and cautioned her to be careful in moving her neck and asked her to wear a cervical collar. The ENT doctor briefed her that audiometry showed significant hearing loss in the ears and said she had peripheral vertigo due to the ear. The neurologist told her that the blood vessels supplying blood to her brain were narrowed and she would have to take a blood thinner for the rest of her life to prevent a stroke.

Overnight, a happy and healthy lady found that she had three problems to live with henceforth: narrowed blood supply to the brain, wear and tear in her cervical spine, and a problem in both ears. After being told that it was all expected at her age, she felt she had suddenly aged by 20 years.

She went home after three days, but would still need some support to walk even within her house. She felt milder but sudden, unpredictable attacks of spinning; sometimes when getting up from bed, sometimes when putting her head on the bed, sometimes when reaching for a jar of sugar, and sometimes on bending down to pick up her slippers.

Around a month later, the attacks stopped, she regained confidence, ventured back to her laughter club, and restarted her earlier routine. She even forgot about her cervical collar and stopped worrying about the blood supply to her brain.

But she got a rude shock two months later, as she got out of bed, felt the room spin, and fell. Luckily, for her, there was no major injury or fracture from the fall.

But the fall and the occasional mild bouts of dizziness shattered her confidence and she stopped going to the laughter club. She now needed someone to get grocery. She was scared to move her neck and started getting pain in her neck due to the collar and the new pillow. She lived in dread of getting paralyzed and could no longer enjoy music as it didn't sound the same anymore.

Mrs B came to see me after three years, after around ten doctors and physiotherapists. She had symptoms every few months and was resigned to a semi-dependent and relatively inactive life, and would take anti-vertigo tablets every now and then and felt this was what her remaining life was to be.

Luckily, after a fresh attack, she was referred to me by someone who had the same experience earlier. She had definite BPPV and we immediately did an Epley repositioning manoeuvre. Mrs B could not believe that within minutes of this simple manoeuvre, her vertigo immediately stopped. All it involved was a set of head and body movements in a sequence to move certain calcium particles in her inner ear, back to where they should have been. She was also advised rehabilitation exercises to gain back her balance and confidence. Within a month, her laughter club and her regular routine were back after a gap of nearly two years. Her joy was all the gratitude we needed.

## Case 3

Mr A, a 50-year-old bank manager, came to see me for sudden unexplained attacks of vertigo, coming out of the blue, unrelated to any head movement. There was also nausea and often vomiting and he would remain lying down in a dark and quiet room for a few hours till he felt better. Sometimes there would be a ringing noise in his ears. Initially, these attacks occurred once in a few months. But now, for the last three months, he was getting them almost every week.

His family doctor had guided him to an ENT surgeon, who found some hearing loss in both ears on audiometry; documented a normal MRI brain, and diagnosed him with Meniere's disease. Mr A googled and found to his dismay that there was no good therapy for Meniere's disease and that he might be doomed to unpredictable attacks indefinitely.

He came to me for a second opinion. He seemed like an anxious person. There was no neurological deficit and his vestibular tests were also normal. The routine screening questionnaire, which he had filled before seeing me, suggested significant anxiety.

His detailed history revealed that Mr A had been getting occasional headaches right from school, but for the last five years, he had rare headaches, for example on missing a meal or if he slept late.

Three years ago he became the manager of his bank. soon thereafter, he started getting attacks of vertigo once or twice a month. Four months ago, he got promoted to regional head of his bank. A month later, he started getting weekly attacks of vertigo.

I diagnosed him with vestibular migraine and explained to him how his vertigo correlated with his stress and increased responsibility at work. I explained to him how migraine is not just a tendency to get headaches, but can also frequently result in attacks of vertigo and dizziness, sometimes independent of headaches.

I prescribed migraine preventive medicines for a few months, asked him to pay attention to stress, learn to cope with and delegate his responsibilities, and start regular exercise, meditation, and have meals on time. In a few months, we were able to get him off all drugs and he only gets rare attacks of milder vertigo.

## Case 4

Mr R, a 42-year-old man, was referred for psychotherapy by his neurologist. He had been to various specialists. His symptoms had started slowly a year ago and gradually worsened. He would feel dizzy, almost every other day, for a few seconds or minutes. Sometimes just a glass of water would help; sometimes, he would have to hold onto a table for support, till the *dizzy wave* passed. He had no problem when driving but strangely would sometimes feel dizzy while waiting at a traffic signal. Sometimes it got worse on head and neck movement; sometimes when working for a long time on the laptop. He saw a physician and when a battery of tests turned out normal, he was asked to see a neurotologist, who diagnosed it as PPPD, prescribed necessary medicine and vestibular rehabilitation, and referred him for CBT.

As a therapist, I found the biopsychosocial model to be the best way forward as his symptoms needed to be monitored from the medical angle as well. I realized that there was great reluctance on the patient's part to accept that stress or some emotional disturbance could be causing or aggravating his 'obviously physical' symptoms.

He preferred to focus completely only the physical distress and spent a great deal of time talking about them. When he realized that I was not judging him, he felt safe and was able to vent his feelings completely. This process of catharsis itself led to a slight reduction in his symptoms and was the beginning of the road to his recovery. He gradually started openly discussing his everyday worries and anxieties. There was not a single major problem. Although his children were growing up beautifully, they were in their teenage years and were going through their own phase of storm and stress. Although his business was expanding steadily, he was faced with difficult decisions almost on a daily basis. His mother had minor age-related health issues and that was always at the back of his mind. These constant undercurrents of anxiety, like white noise, kept him on his toes and never really allowed him to be at ease for long. As the days passed, a pattern slowly emerged and became visible not only to me as his therapist but to him too. He also realized that the dizziness was his mind's way of asking for a break from the endless loop of anxious thoughts.

This opened the doors to the next stage of therapy. The best way to break the maladaptive pattern was to examine each distressing thought and change it to a healthier one. This is how cognitive restructuring was achieved. All the situations and events remained the same, but he learnt more adaptive ways to deal with them. A balanced nutritious diet, adequate exercise, and six weeks of psychotherapy helped the patient to regain his confidence, overcome the PPPD, and lead a comfortable life. Although he had relapses now and then, his therapy tools helped him to identify and overcome the triggers.

## Case 5

Another case that comes to mind is of Mrs J. A 38-year-old IT professional. Mrs J was on her way home from grocery shopping when her two-wheeler went out of control and ended up with her on the road, face down, pinned by the vehicle. It was only a split second later that she realized she was surrounded by people. Some curious bystanders, some genuinely helpful people. Someone lifted her bike while someone else helped her sit by the side of the road. A rickshaw driver became a good Samaritan and ferried her to the nearest hospital. She called up her husband who rushed to meet her at the casualty department.

After a thorough examination by the orthopaedic doctor at the casualty, she was told that she had been extremely lucky as she had only sustained minor injuries on her ankle. No head injuries and no other trauma. She left the hospital shaken and exhausted from the events of the day. The painkillers prescribed by the doctor at the hospital helped with the pain but she slept fitfully that night. She had recurring dreams about the accident and the nameless faces that kept peering at her as she lay on the road. The whole incident kept replaying in her mind. The next morning, as she got out of bed, she felt a sudden dizziness that caught her off guard. As she steadied herself, a sense of dread overcame her. What if the doctor had missed something? What if there was something truly amiss? She had to get back to the hospital immediately. She got dressed and spoke to her husband about her dizziness. He was concerned too. They requested an urgent appointment with the same doctor they had seen the previous day. He recommended that they see a neurologist instead. Mrs J found herself in the neurology wing of the hospital a short while later. The senior consultant was not available and the resident on call recommended she get an MRI scan right away. Mrs J knew something was wrong.

While undergoing the scan, she couldn't stop thinking about her accident. She had fallen quite badly. She knew this dizziness was not something she had experienced before. She tried to understand the nature of the dizziness to try and explain it to the senior doctor when she saw him next. It was intermittent. But it was distressing. She had to be vigilant. After all, it was her health, and she had to take responsibility. The MRI scan luckily turned out to be normal. Her appointment with the neurologist was fixed for the end of the week.

Mrs J was sure her symptoms were worsening. She was dizzy in the shower sometimes. Sometimes it would hit her when she was out with her family in the car. The resident had asked her to watch out for any increase in the frequency or intensity of the episodes. And they were getting worse. By the time the day of the appointment came, she was debilitated by the dizziness. It made her feel anxious and she was scared to go anywhere alone. Her husband helped her sit gingerly in the chair and they both seemed tired as they spoke to the consultant. When the doctor saw the scans and examined the patient clinically, he recommended a psychiatric consult to deal with probable post traumatic stress disorder or PTSD first. He assured Mrs J that he would reevaluate her symptoms after the psychiatrist had seen and started treatment.

Mrs J was open to the idea and met the psychiatrist as soon as the appointment was given. She was diagnosed to have PPPD resulting from PTSD. The psychiatrist started her on a prescription for the PTSD and recommended therapy after six weeks. It was a combination of the drugs and therapy that helped her deal effectively with the post-traumatic stress. Her dizziness eased as a consequence of the treatment too. When she saw the neurologist after eight weeks, she had been free of the dizziness for a few days and was optimistic that the remission would be a long-lasting one.

Various triggers can lead to PPPD. Sometimes life situations and micro stressors can build up, leading to this kind of dizziness. Sometimes there can be a single clear precipitating factor, like a physical trauma/accident, or an intense life event. While most doctors believe that a certain personality type (the anxious or hyper-vigilant ones) are more likely to suffer from PPPD, it has been seen to occur in almost all personality types. Treatment can literally be learning to live a balanced life.

# CHAPTER 8
# Tinnitus: Ring out the Old

~With Dr Milind Kirtane
and Dr Jaini Lodha Bhandari

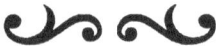

Tinnitus is a common complaint where the person hears a ringing or hissing noise in one or both ears. It is only in their brain-mind; no one else hears it. It is disturbing and distressing and affects people's quality of life. It used to be considered essentially a disorder of the ear, but now, increasingly, the role of the brain-mind is being realized.

Sound consists of vibrations passing through the air, reaching the ear, where they are amplified and converted into electrical signals, and taken to the brain, which perceives the sound, and makes meaning out of it, be it music or voice or words. Since these vibrations reach the other's ears, they can also hear this sound.

There are some psychiatric and brain disorders, called auditory hallucinations, where a person hears imaginary persons talking to them or may hear music. Tinnitus also is 'imaginary' in that no one else hears it, but unlike hallucinations, there are no formed words or musical instruments; it is just unformed sounds like a whistle, hiss, hum, or buzz.

Tinnitus is quite common with increasing age, with a prevalence ranging from 10% to 15%. In most of these, it fades off. But in 1–2% people it can disrupt sleep, interfere with concentration, and cause emotional and mood disturbances, and does not allow the person to enjoy a normal social life.

Like many other functional disorders, the suffering is worse because they do not have anything to show for it; no scar, plaster, bandage, wheelchair. It is just a sound in one's head, which no one else hears, and so others may not believe, understand, or have any empathy for the sufferer.

In general, if the tinnitus is not associated with hearing loss or is faint and heard only at night or when it is quiet all around, it is unlikely to be significant. On the other hand, if it associated with significant hearing loss; and bothers the person when he/she is talking to others or is at work, it needs evaluation.

## How does tinnitus develop?

Tinnitus is essentially a faulty attempt of the brain to make up for a loss of hearing. The loss of hearing may be due to damage anywhere in the hearing pathway, right from the ear to the brain. The commonest site is the ear wax, infection in the middle ear, or damage to the delicate inner ear hair cells by exposure to excessively loud noises.

Impaired hearing due to any cause leads to less sound information reaching the brain. Like an amplifier, the brain turns up the volume to try and hear whatever little comes through. In this attempt, it may end up creating a sound where there is none, namely tinnitus. This sound matches the missing tone. Like with any skill, once the brain 'learns' tinnitus, it does not forget it easily. Tinnitus persists even if you cut the nerve from the ear to the brain. To treat tinnitus, we have to target the brain as well as the ear.

After an initial ear injury, the brain habituates and tinnitus dies out in most people. But, in a small percentage of people, the tinnitus persists and becomes chronic. Who are these persons who are unable to turn down the volume? As it turns out, it is precisely the ones who get more worried, more irritated, annoyed or bothered by the sound. How a person reacts to or adapts to a hearing loss or tinnitus may depend on his personality and psychological profile. Tinnitus can worsen anxiety and depression, leading to a vicious circle.

Thus, though the original trigger is usually some organic ear disorder, long term suffering is usually due to psychological factors. In many ways, tinnitus is like chronic pain and the phenomenon of central sensitization.

## How do we manage tinnitus?

In a nutshell, we need to correct the loss of hearing as far as possible. If the person can learn to live with the remaining hearing loss and not feel threatened or bothered by the tinnitus, it often abates.

The first and most important step is to try to improve hearing. If that is not possible, even a hearing aid or a device to create a masking sound can help.

The second step is to reduce anxiety, fear, and memory. Psycho-education may help in reducing anxiety, while CBT can help in reducing the annoyance and irritation. Simple questionnaires can tell us how much the person is bothered by the tinnitus. If it is mild, just a little reassurance may be all that is needed. Those who are disabled significantly, need a team approach with an ENT surgeon, audiologist, and a CBT trainer or psychologist.

## *Case 1*

By Dr Kirtane

My dear friend Dr (Mr) ABC, who walked into my OPD casually one busy Saturday afternoon, saying that he had some sound in his head, which started all of a sudden that morning. He had a common cold attack a few days ago, other than this he had no positive history of loud noise exposure or head injury or dizziness. I sent him to get an audiometry test (hearing test) done, which was normal. Well, I passed it off casually and just counselled him to ignore the noise and sleep well over the weekend and relax. Again, after a week of seeing him, next Monday morning I saw him waiting anxiously outside my cabin even before my OPD started. His ringing noise in the ear had now become like a screeching noise in the ear and he had not slept for four nights straight. He was so visibly stressed that he had tremors and had cancelled all his scheduled surgeries in the operating theatre. I realized that this had to be dealt with compassion and patient listening. On detailed history taking, I realized that Dr ABC lost his beloved mother in a car accident a couple of months ago. He was a single father trying to cope with his mother's loss and bringing up his son single-handedly, to add to that his work commitments and busy schedule at the hospital had left him overburdened, stressed, and grieving. We eventually gave him tinnitus retraining therapy (TRT), psychological counselling, and counselled him to engage himself in a hobby he likes. He was a fighter and decided to take this challenge head-on, and till date, he is coping well with his struggles, his tinnitus is fairly under control with intermittent periods of aggravation, which he has learnt to get in control with relaxation therapies."

## Conclusion

Thus we have seen how tinnitus is a maladaptive attempt by the brain (and mind) to make up for the hearing loss. Once we have corrected the hearing loss as best as we can, helping the patient to relax, accept, and live with it, is the way that the sound will stop tormenting them.

# CHAPTER 9

# Pulmonology: Breathe in, Breathe out

~With Dr Sanjeev Mehta

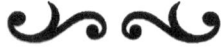

Somehow, when I was asked to share my experiences with patients with psychosomatic manifestations, the first word that hit me was *inspire* – a term that has both respiratory and psychological connotations. Funnily enough, there are even statements such as: "I need my breathing space," - which imply the need for freedom – another expression connecting breath to the mind. We are often told to take a deep breath whenever we are nervous; for example, before facing a crowd, performing on stage, giving an examination, and the like. Surprisingly, this simple activity does help calm the mind. Breathing is considered an extremely vital part of life. We all have gasped on seeing a baby take his first breath or possibly someone breathe his last.

The fact that the body and the mind work in unison and affect each other practically all the time has been known since ancient times; however, its implications in clinical practice are increasingly being recognized by the medical fraternity now. In fact, over 2500 years ago, Socrates had reprimanded the physicians of his time for their overly organic medical attitude. He advocated holistic healing and firmly believed that the body could not be completely cured without treating the mind.

Aristotle went a step further to say that emotions had a direct impact on physiologic processes and this was generally the prevailing idea till the rise of dualistic thinking in the seventeenth century.

Again, in the latter half of the nineteenth century, the French neurologist Charcot used hypnotism to treat certain physical symptoms of psychic origin, for example, hysterical seizures. Influenced by him, Freud took the baton forward, reinstated the therapeutic doctor-patient relationship, and envisioned the potential role of psychotherapy in the management of certain patients. Despite so much evidence against it, dualistic thinking still resides deep within the mind of many, laymen as well as doctors.

## Psychosomatic elements of respiratory diseases

It is not at all surprising, that disorders of breathing can be a symptom of a psychosomatic disorder. We know how important breathing is for health. Life starts and ends with a breath and multiple religions associate breath with spirit. The lexicon used in everyday expressions is overlapping too. 'Breathing a sigh of relief'; 'took my breath away', etc. are just a few commonly used phrases indicating this overlap.

As humans, we take involuntary functions of our body for granted most of the time, except – of course – when something goes wrong. We hardly ever realize that breathing plays a vital role not only in keeping us alive by oxygenating the body cells, but also when expressing emotions by way of laughter or crying.

Our breathing also reflects our state of mind. We are aware of the effect of our state of mind on our breathing; jerky shallow breathing when anxious or angry, slow and deep breathing when relaxed. Even the pattern of breathing, whether predominantly abdominal or thoracic varies.

What is interesting is the effect of breathing on our state of mind. Breathing is the link between the involuntary and voluntary nervous systems and is one of the rare activities, which are under the control of both. For example, we can choose to purposely hold our breath for some time or can breathe harder or faster, if we choose to. In fact, one of the commonest ways of meditation involves watching one's breath and allowing it to settle down. This seems to calm the mind. It can be as simple as taking a deep breath or counting to 10 slowly or it can be elaborate like the special breathing techniques of Yoga and Pranayama.

## *Psychosomatic respiratory disorders*

The common respiratory symptoms which can be psychosomatic are disorders of breathing, a dry cough, a change in voice or chest pain. Like with the other psychosomatic disorders, one cannot find any respiratory disorder to explain them or even if there is a disorder, the symptoms are clearly out of proportion and excessive. The symptoms may be atypical for that disorder or may not be responding to appropriate therapy.

There are two basic scenarios to be considered.

The first situation is when the disorder develops in isolated association with a clear psychological stressor. For example, sudden stridor and difficulty breathing in a young athlete before an important event; or loss of voice before an interview or exam. The relation to the stressor is obvious. This is not such a common situation and may respond to behavioural and psychological treatments alone.

The more common situation is when symptoms get aggravated inexplicably in a person with a known respiratory disorder. It may happen after some stress or maybe anxiety after getting exposed to dust. These require a combination of medical management for the respiratory disorder, plus attention to the anxiety or stressor.

In order to understand the psychosomatic elements of respiratory diseases, one needs to appreciate the integrated operations of the respiratory system, central nervous system, and the mind. Patients suffering from severe anxiety often report experiencing other symptoms such as light-headedness, giddiness, faintness, and blurring of vision; almost all of which can be replicated by asking the patient to hyperventilate or breathe hard and excessively on purpose.

Bronchial asthma, an important psycho-physiological respiratory disorder, gives rise to various signs and symptoms as a result of intermittent episodes of bronchial obstruction that is usually reversible in character. This disease is multifactorial in origin, i.e. no single etiologic determinant has been specifically labelled as the only culprit. Various allergic, endocrine, genetic, infectious, psychological, and social factors are there to blame, but not one of them exclusively rules the roost. There is a growing body of evidence to show that several cases of asthma are triggered by or aggravated by psychological factors.

Investigators who attempted to establish associations between chronic obstructive pulmonary disease (COPD) and other respiratory disorders, and a person's psychological state, have drawn up various findings. Although a single psychological state cannot be pointed at with regards to a specific respiratory disorder, there is no denying that overlaps are common and that finding out what is truly causing the symptoms can be detrimental in finding the most effective treatment plan.

The truth is that the level of dyspnea, or shortness of breath, varies in the same person at different points in time and under differing circumstances. Further, while dyspnea could be an outward manifestation of any emotional stress, it can be caused by an underlying cardiopulmonary disorder; and the symptom by itself can be distressing enough to produce great anxiety and fear. Practically all patients with dyspnea, depending on the severity of their breathlessness and availability of the doctor, are likely to consult a general physician, pulmonologist, or cardiologist, rather than a psychiatrist. Therefore, every physician must also keep psychogenic dyspnea at the back of his or her mind, when contemplating on the differential diagnoses of a breathless patient. Three variations of psychogenic dyspnea should be considered, namely anxious breathing or panic attacks, psychogenic hyperventilation syndrome, and compulsive sighing.

The respiratory subtype of panic attacks is a manifestation of acute anxiety and is characterized by shallow and irregular breathing, which is mostly thoracic and not abdominal. The onset may be rapid or gradual, and the patient may also complain of symptoms such as giddiness, palpitations, and tremors that usually subside on their own. An increased sensitivity to $CO_2$ is seen in these cases, and a family history of panic disorders can often be elicited. Brought on by a surge of adrenaline into the bloodstream, this is a type of *fight or flight response* that allows for increased oxygenation of tissues by raising the respiratory rate and blood pressure. Normal people experience this phenomenon too, the only difference being that it lasts for a very short period. However, in patients with panic attacks, the entire episode gets prolonged and leads to variable signs and symptoms. Initially, the patient may only experience dizziness, palpitations, and sweating. In the intermediate stages, she/he may complain of abdominal distress, chills, chest pain, choking, dyspnea, nausea, and trembling. In the later stages, the patient may develop a fear of going crazy or fear of dying. Paresthesias are also common in this stage, along with a sense of altered reality.

Psychogenic hyperventilation syndrome is an attention-seeking behavioural condition that is triggered by acute emotional stress. It is easy to recognize, once a physician has come across a case in his or her clinical practice. Such patients generally complain of sudden onset of severe breathlessness. There may be associated symptoms like giddiness, extreme fatigue, finger contractions, and tinnitus. At times, mild tachycardia may be detected. Some organic causes of hyperventilation such as acute myocardial infarction, brainstem stroke, carbon monoxide poisoning, foreign body aspiration, pulmonary embolism, and tension pneumothorax can also trigger the very same cascade of metabolic events. In majority of the cases, these can be ruled out based on the history and examination findings. Investigations may be required only in a small number of cases. Getting the patient to breathe in a paper bag suffices to reverse the cascade and restore normalcy by increasing the $CO_2$ levels in the blood. However, this should ideally be followed by sessions of cognitive-behavioural therapy.

Compulsive sighing is basically a clinical diagnosis and is characterized by recurrent, forced deep inhalations followed by a prolonged sigh that is often audible. Involuntary sighing up to eight times per hour is normal; but when this becomes frequent, it becomes a problem. The patient usually feels that his or her breath is incomplete, despite sighing. Respiration is otherwise shallow, and a precipitating cause cannot be pinpointed;

as these episodes occur spontaneously and last for variable periods of time, ranging from a few days to weeks or months. Although this happens more often in solitude and at rest, it does not occur during sleep. The patient's speech remains unaltered, and physical activity does not worsen the sighing in any manner. An old, suppressed, and unresolved negative emotion is usually the cause in patients with this sigh syndrome.

Psychogenic breathing can easily be differentiated from dyspnea due to organic causes. The former is more prominent at rest but absent during sleep. Typical environmental triggers are absent. Probing into the mind space of the patient often reveals the presence of an underlying emotional traumatic event. Above all, the results of diagnostic tests are almost always normal. The good thing is that the conscious mind can be taught to experience dyspnea to a lesser extent. This offers a therapeutic advantage, not only in cases of psychogenic dyspnea but also when there is a respiratory condition in the background. The patient feels better even if the underlying pathology has remained unchanged. This is precisely why psychosomatic medicine has an important role to play in the treatment of all diseases. Ideally, some doctors feel, it should be recommended as a supplementary therapy in each and every patient, as this could help reduce the number of medications being prescribed and thereby decrease the incidence of iatrogenic diseases. Another important point is that everything is not black or white. There are always shades of grey in between. Similarly, diseases like asthma can definitely overlap and coexist with panic attacks and hyperventilation syndrome. Hence, the presence of one does not preclude the existence of the other.

A missed diagnosis or a wrong diagnosis often leaves both the patient and physician fuming or flustered. Having witnessed several interesting cases in my clinical practice, I am sharing two such cases that are in context. They are important from the standpoint of learning from our own or others' mistakes. The value of being logical and methodical when arriving at a diagnosis and before enthusiastic pharmacological management is emphasized on in the first case. In the second case, the exact opposite is noted, where an erroneous diagnosis led to a delay in appropriate treatment and has been associated with adverse outcomes.

## Case 1

It was a warm Sunday afternoon, and I was relaxing on my couch watching television, when I received a call from my hospital. It was the houseman on duty on the other end, who told me that there was an emergency and I was needed. Tulsi (name changed to maintain anonymity), a 17-year-old girl had been brought into the casualty by her mother, who was visibly upset by her daughter's plight. The houseman had observed that she was in a diaphoretic state and was breathing rapidly and deeply. She had her hand on her chest, as she complained of a sense of pressure. She also said that her head was aching, and her vision had blurred. On examination, her heart rate was found to be slightly higher at 94 beats/minute; but chest auscultation revealed no abnormality.

The mother revealed that they stayed in a village that was about 150 km away from the city. This was the eighth time that the girl had experienced this breathlessness, and hence, her mother had taken help from a neighbour to bring her to the city hospital. Her past episodes had been managed in a local primary care centre, where the doctor had assumed that the patient was asthmatic and managed her with supplemental oxygen and inhaled β2-adrenergic bronchodilators. Since her second episode was apparently worse than the first, a corticosteroid had also been administered orally at the time.

The workup in the emergency department included various investigations, namely a complete blood cell count, thyroid screening, electrocardiography, chest X-ray, arterial blood gases, and serum levels of electrolytes, bicarbonate, calcium, and magnesium. All the diagnostic tests reported normal, except for the arterial blood gases report, which was slightly abnormal with a pH of 7.51, $pCO_2$ of 32 mmHg, and $pO_2$ of 99 mmHg in room air. Even spirometry detected nothing abnormal.

Probing further into this patient's history showed that the previous episodes had occurred spontaneously on different occasions, such as in school, at home, in the marketplace, and in a friend's or neighbour's house. She never had these episodes at night or when she was alone. All these years, in between episodes, she had never been completely well. Frequent headaches and abdominal queasiness were common issues along with shortness of breath, which she experienced on a regular basis. She usually found relief by sitting in front of a table fan.

When I got there, my houseman had kept all the details of the case ready and had initiated symptomatic treatment. However, he confided in me and said that she was not responding to the bronchodilator therapy even in a high dose. In fact, she claimed to be getting worse and 'shaky' with the treatment. He was a young doctor who was apprehensive, as he couldn't think of a diagnosis; but having come across such patients in the past and knowing that this girl had been treated only by the local village doctors, I asked everyone present there to stay calm, whispered into the houseman's ears to stop all medications, and messaged my psychiatrist friend to pay a visit.

I deliberately told my friend not to reveal her specialty to the patient and her mother. She was to simply talk to this girl as just another doctor. There were too many pointers to indicate a functional respiratory disorder: her normal oxygen saturation, mild alkalosis, normal examination and investigatory findings, non-response to bronchodilator therapy, the occurrence of episodes only in the presence of others and never at night or in her sleep, and her ability to frankly verbalize and/or take oral medications during respiratory distress.

Most patients with functional causes of dyspnea are asymptomatic when asleep at night and when distracted in the day time. They are capable of talking fluently during an episode. On the other hand, patients with organic causes of severe dyspnea can hardly say a few words – that too – with great difficulty. The mild respiratory alkalosis is not something to be alarmed about, as it is the consequence of acute hyperventilation, an established component of panic disorders or chronic anxiety. My gut feeling was proved right by my friend who interviewed the girl and her mother separately after some medical histrionics from our side had relieved the patient. Placebo pills and an injection of vitamin B-complex had been administered to the girl, and she was asked to breathe wearing a facemask that had no oxygen supply in it, so as to get her to inhale the air exhaled by her to increase the $CO_2$ level. She responded beautifully.

Although I was a bit amused about the whole matter initially, I was left completely shaken and teary-eyed after I learned more about this patient from my psychiatrist friend. She revealed that the girl and her mother hailed from a very backward region in India. To make matters worse, they belonged to an extremely conservative family, which firmly believed that females are a lower species and also a burden on their parents. Female foeticide and infanticide were fearlessly and shamelessly practised in their community. Years ago, the girl had overheard her mother speaking to a relative about how her husband had tried to get her aborted after finding out illegally that a daughter was going to be born, but destiny had something else in store.

In the patient's infancy, her father had tried to smother her with a pillow. When he was caught red-handed by his wife, he painted a sorry picture and apologized. All seemed okay till the girl was five years-old. The family had gone for an outing near a lake, when the father pushed the girl into the water, well aware that she did not know swimming and would drown. The patient was lucky again, as some passerby saw her drowning, jumped in, and saved her life. The girl could sense that her father was pretending to be good in the presence of others and was showing his true colours only when he was alone with her. These events had subconsciously affected the patient to such an extent that she had become claustrophobic and feared becoming breathless.

At seven years of age, her father found an opportunity to get rid of her again. With his parents and wife having gone to attend a funeral, he asked his daughter to take a bath, forced her to use the smallest bathroom in their house, and locked the door from outside. The girl's hapless screams failed to melt his stone heart. She cried herself sore and eventually fainted. The patient's mother had an inkling about her husband's evil intentions; so, she had excused herself from the rites early and returned home, only to find her daughter unconscious. This was when she realized that the Damocles' sword was still dangling over her child's neck. After a lot of thinking, she gathered all her courage and escaped with her daughter to come and stay with her aunt, who had always been very supportive. Ten years had passed, but their emotional wounds were fresh as ever.

The mother had braved the separation with fortitude, but the daughter remained anxious and fearful. Her intensity of breathlessness kept varying, and she had a lot of associated symptoms as well, but none of the primary healthcare doctors had realized that she was a case of psychogenic dyspnea. Now, after several sessions of psychotherapy, the girl is much better; although she says that she continues to have nightmares of being drowned, throttled, smothered, or getting choked. Overall, her sense of well-being seems to be returning, and her self-esteem is definitely on the rise. Whenever I think of this case, my hair stands on end; and I shudder to think about what could have happened if the mother had not taken the bold step of dumping her husband to protect her child. The entire story felt so dramatic that I couldn't believe that it had actually come to pass.

## Case 2

This is one of my other memorable cases, as it had reminded me of 'the boy who cried wolf' from Aesop's fables, where frequent false alarms raised by a boy got people so immune to his shouts for help, that they failed to turn up when a wolf really came along, and his call was genuine. This 20-year-old college student named Vivek (name changed to maintain anonymity) had come with his parents to the hospital that I was attached to as an honorary consultant. They were completely unaware of my presence there and were taken aback on seeing me, as I had treated this boy six years ago when they had come to my private clinic.

Aged 14 at that time, he used to cough so loudly that it irritated everyone around him. His parents had received complaints from his school teachers that he needed to be treated properly, as his cough disrupted the class often. His problem had apparently started a year earlier after having suffered from a severe upper respiratory tract infection, along with high-grade fever. The purulence of his sputum had aroused suspicion of a streptococcal throat; and therefore, a five-day antibiotic course had been prescribed for him by his family physician. Although he recovered from the illness, his cough seemed to have persisted since then. It was typically barking in nature, and the patient assumed a characteristic 'chin-on-chest' posture whenever he coughed.

He had no expectoration, breathlessness, fatigue, or voice change. I had got him investigated thoroughly then, but all his reports were normal. Initially, I did try various medicines to relieve him, right from antihistamines and decongestants to antitussives; but soon I realized the futility of this exercise, considering that this boy never responded to anything. I stopped and advised his parents to consult a psychiatrist, as I strongly felt that his problem was psychogenic. He was probably a case of habit cough. I took them into confidence and explained the pathogenesis of cough in such cases. Few hints had been dropped in by the parents themselves, who disclosed that their lad was full of insecurities and was suffering from an inferiority complex; because his elder brother outshone him in every way – looks, studies, sports, style, talent, habits, and manners. Full of jealousy, the patient had been indulging in attention-seeking behaviour from early childhood. In fact, he stopped wetting the bed at the age of 12 years. He did not want to share anything with his sibling.

I had clearly told the boy's parents to follow-up with me at regular intervals and to keep me informed about his progress, even when he was undergoing psychotherapy; but I have no idea as to what they were thinking at that time. They never showed up again. Now, after a period of six years, they were looking into my eyes with mixed emotions: guilt, sadness, expectations, and what not. They revealed that they had indeed visited a psychiatrist after I had told them to do so, and the latter had confirmed the diagnosis of habit cough. Unfortunately, they did not know the importance of psychotherapy in such cases and gave it up after just a few sessions. Once they understood that their son was physically healthy and his cough was emotional in origin, they chose to ignore the symptom, not realizing that they were feeding his insecurities further in the bargain.

He had gradually started to withdraw socially. He wasn't eating well, and his parents again thought that he was being fussy. In the last two years, his cough had progressively worsened; and he complained of shortness of breath and fatigue off and on. Every time he cribbed about his problems, it only made his parents more irritable, as they felt that he was pretending or giving excuses to avoid running errands, to shirk his responsibilities, or to bunk his classes. Despite realizing that he was possibly sinking into depression, the parents continued to nag him with the hope that he would mend his ways; but what forced them to rush with him to the hospital this time was something that had scared the hell out of them. That morning, after a bout of cough, the boy spat out blood into the washbasin and was conspicuously breathless. The whole house was in a state of panic, as they knew that this could not be a part of his emotional problem. His mother was in tears and his father was full of remorse. They literally begged me for help and were prepared to do anything to salvage the situation. I asked them to stay calm, admitted the patient, and ordered a battery of tests for the boy.

His chest X-ray showed consolidation of the middle and lower lobe of the right lung, along with blunting of the right costophrenic angle, which was suggestive of pleural effusion. A culture of his sputum grew *Streptococcus pyogenes* that was sensitive to piperacillin and tazobactam. His sputum sample also tested positive for the presence of *Mycobacterium tuberculosis*. He was thus a case of active pulmonary Koch's disease with secondary infection. Involvement of the bronchial artery had led to hemoptysis in this case. Contrast-enhanced computerized tomography of the thorax was performed to assess the state of the lung better. Multiple cavities were found to have developed in the afflicted area and there was large scale damage to the pulmonary architecture.

The patient was immediately put on antibiotics and antitubercular treatment. In order to offer symptomatic relief, the excess pleural fluid was also drained. Although I knew that the boy would be fine, I was also aware that with so much of lung involvement, the scar that would eventually remain was certainly going to predispose chronic lung disease. If only the parents had not neglected the boy's symptoms and presumed that they were psychogenic, things could have been very different. An early diagnosis of tuberculosis would obviously have been followed by prompt treatment, and the prevention of such complications. This boy improved and went home with a smile on his face, but I had to inform the parents that things would never be completely normal again. Although he was symptomatically much better, spirometry continued to show a restrictive pattern due to pulmonary fibrosis. Thus, he could comfortably attend to his routine, but any form of physical overexertion was likely to make him breathless again.

It is very important for both laymen as well as physicians to always keep an open mind. Just because an individual has been diagnosed with a certain disease due to the presence of a particular set of symptoms, does not mean that other diseases with a similar set of symptoms cannot concur in the same person. The frequent association between respiratory disorders and psychiatric illnesses is not surprising at all, considering that breathing and emotions are bidirectionally related. It is quite intriguing that breathing is the first sign of life and the psyche becomes active only at birth. In some cases, respiratory symptoms can be the only indication of a psychological conflict. Psychogenic respiratory disorders often mimic organic conditions and trigger a cascade of diagnostic and therapeutic interventions that cost the patient his or her money as well as mental peace. Hence, a prudent clinician should know how to recognize these patients from their history and examination findings. Long-term psychotherapy is needed to produce lasting improvement. Therefore, educating the patient and his or her family members is an absolute must.

# CHAPTER 10

# Orthopaedics: A Bone to Pick

~With Dr Sandeep Patwardhan

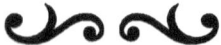

Pain is one of the most common manifestations of psychosomatic illness. Pain in the neck, back or limbs and joints comprise many patients. The doctor does think of a psychological cause when the pain is in multiple areas, keeps shifting from one site to another, or is vague and poorly localized. It is a fallacy though to not consider psychological factors when the pain affects a single region, like the back or neck or one limb or one joint. It is not uncommon for these pains to get pinned onto a minor aberration or 'abnormality'. In addition, we should not forget the role of psychological factors in impeding recovery from definite injuries or joint problems.

Sometimes, when a person refers to pain in a certain limb or back/neck, he or she adds voluntarily that the pain is not allowing them to do certain work. For example, someone with chronic pain in the wrist may be unable to do household chores while someone with severe chronic backache might be more likely to leave the office early to avoid sitting for long hours. This immediate gain can make it seem like the patient is 'using' their pain for an ulterior gain.

What is important from the doctor's perspective is to understand that malingering is the exception and not the norm. Most patients presenting with such pains are not suffering voluntarily. They have real pain and need treatment. This treatment may not be mainstream orthopaedic in nature and might need intervention from a mental health specialist, but that does not make the pain unreal or the patient a malingerer.

## Fibromyalgia

Fibromyalgia has been a very disputed disorder, with controversies about every aspect of it, including the existence, cause, pathophysiology, diagnosis, and treatment. It is very common, affecting 1–5% of the population, and is the second most common musculoskeletal condition after osteoarthritis.

Basically, the person has unexplained chronic widespread pains. There are no abnormal findings on any test and yet this is real pain and not malingering. Of course, it is not uncommon that some minor abnormality gets blamed and the diagnosis gets delayed for years.

Apart from widespread muscular and joint pains, there is often fatigue, poor sleep, impaired memory, and depression. It is now accepted that fibromyalgia is a functional disorder with abnormal processing of pain signals leading to sensitization or amplification of pain. Functional brain imaging has shown that the person feels more pain for a given stimulus than a normal person. It often coexists with other pain syndromes, like irritable bowel syndrome or migraine headaches, sometimes in families. It seems to happen due to a combination of genetic predisposition, triggered by trauma, acute stress, or illness.

The diagnosis no longer needs a doctor to examine and document tender or painful areas on the body. Instead, just a history of widespread pain for over three months is enough to diagnose it. The diagnosis is now made positively and not by ruling out various causes and not finding anything else, finally declaring it is fibromyalgia.

Making a diagnosis helps both the patient and the doctor deal with it effectively. It ends the anxiety and uncertainty and helps reduce unnecessary tests and consultations. It helps being open about the multi-focal approach that is most effective in treating fibromyalgia. When patients accept at the outset that along with medical treatment and physiotherapy, they will also benefit from psychotherapy, the results are usually much better.

## Neck pain and back pain

They are commonly psychosomatic in origin. Almost 4–5 adults will have significant back pain sometime during their life, with most recovering within weeks without any specific treatment. The causes include poor posture, lack of exercise, stress, vitamin deficiency, and degeneration of the spine, and various emotional factors.

As the pain is specific and localized, emotional factors are easily overlooked and various investigations are undertaken to identify the cause of the pain. More often than not, a minor incidental finding takes centre stage and the focus then lies solely on correcting that 'defect' in whatever way possible.

It is natural to feel some distress with pain. But severe pain or chronic pain may often have a great deal of emotional reactions. The pain may induce fear about the possible cause. There can be anxiety as to when and whether the pain will get relieved or not. Pain can also lead to fatigue, both mental and physical. There have been instances when people have complained about being tired despite being on complete rest due to a fractured foot! This fatigue is counter-intuitive as the patient did nothing that would make him or her tired. It is just the constant pain that requires attention and renders the person suffering from it exhausted.

Sometimes, one is scared by finding some abnormality on an MRI or x-ray. They may not be reassured that the finding is innocuous or not related to the pain or not serious in any way. Just being told your joints show wear and tear can scare a person. The person needs to be reassured and told that almost everyone at the person's age shows some wear and tear and the degree of wear and tear is quite normal and not alarming, and is not the cause of the pain. I have seen many people with mild neck or back pain due to some overwork or stress, getting an x-ray or MRI done, and then getting labelled as 'spondylosis' by their doctor. Now they start behaving like a patient of spondylosis and soon start getting all the symptoms they know a person of spondylosis is *supposed* to get. They stop using pillows to sleep or sleep on the floor and end up aggravating their pain.

It can be quite disconcerting and scary to be told by the doctor or friends and relatives that you need to be careful of your back or spine.

You start doubting every activity, stop going to the gym, start limiting your movements and activity, which leads to physical deconditioning and weakness of muscles. This itself perpetuates the back pain.

It is important not to push a patient into this vicious cycle or actively prevent him/her from going into this cycle. Once the patient gets labelled and becomes a chronic patient, it is very difficult to convince him/her that the neck pain was never due to spondylosis. He/she has become a spondylosis patient for life and will go to another doctor, thinking you don't know the diagnosis.

## Arthralgias

Many persons have just vague joint pains without any signs of inflammation and yet get wrongly labelled as chronic arthritis, just because of some blood test coming abnormal once. Psychosomatic factors are very common here.

## Chronic pain due to orthopaedic causes

Various orthopaedic disorders present with chronic pain, including arthritis or spondylosis. All chronic pains are known to get worsened by stress and emotional factors as we already saw in the chapter on pain. Just because the person has a clear underlying cause for pain may lead one to not pay attention to the emotional aspects. In these cases, although stress has not caused the pain, it is playing an important part in aggravating the same.

## Activity limitation and pain

In the early stages of any injury or surgery, one needs to immobilize the area and so rest is very important. Unfortunately, later when the person starts moving, he may get some pain and may wrongly think he is harming his body and avoid that movement. He may substitute that movement with another. Sensitization by the nervous system amplifies his pain signals and so even minor movements, which are not causing any damage, end up causing a lot of pain. This pain scares the patient. The patient needs to understand the pain so he doesn't fear it.

Gradual return to normal movements is crucial for full recovery. There is a concept of bad pain, which signifies tissue injury and which should be avoided. But there is also a good pain, which is the pain that happens when the person fights back against the injury and starts to reclaim back all his normal movements. The difference can be difficult for the patient to understand by himself and so may need to be guided by a physiotherapist and doctor.

Persons who have got into this pain-stress-pain cycle often need multi-disciplinary treatment, including a doctor who makes a confident and firm diagnosis and communicates it clearly to the patient, a physiotherapist and, sometimes, a psychologist. Anti-depressants may sometimes be used to get out of the pain cycle. This is called the biopsychosocial model of treatment. It is very effective in orthopaedic pain management as the medical and psychological aspects are given equal importance, while also considering the social and environmental factors.

## Psychological impact of injuries

Let us also consider the effect of an actual injury on the mind. Let us for example look at a person, who actually suffers an injury to his limb, maybe a fracture of the hip or knee. Such a major fracture would severely affect the ability of the patient to walk unaided and affect his/her day to day life. Often the person would become dependent on others partly or totally, for days, weeks, or even months and years. This can trigger embarrassment, anger, and depression among other feelings. Amputations are an extreme case scenario as they lead to a complete change in a person's body image and need intensive rehabilitation, physically and emotionally.

Sports injuries are another group of injuries which can have a lot of impact on the person's mind. We need to understand that the person's self-esteem and image of himself or herself, and his/her whole career depends on how well he/she plays the sport. If an injury damages, or even threatens to ruin his ability to excel in the sport, it could cause a lot of psychological effects.

Also, some activities like running, give the person a psychological 'high'. If an injury suddenly makes the person stop running, then he is not only deprived of the 'high' but may actually land up in a depression.

To summarize, pain in the back or limbs may often be psychosomatic and be wrongly blamed on a minor abnormality found on testing or imaging. Similarly, actual orthopaedic ailments and injuries can definitely have a major impact on a person's mental and emotional well-being.

## *Case 1*

A pleasant 72-year-old gentleman, Mr Saraf, came to see me yesterday with a note from a rheumatologist, who wanted me to investigate a suspected nerve problem. He was accompanied by his equally pleasant wife.

Like usual, I asked him what was his symptom and since when he had been experiencing it. Mr Saraf started by telling me: "I have been getting pain in the veins of my hands, pointing to the backside of his fingers and palms, as well as well the soles of my feet for the last two years." He went on, "I was diagnosed to have arthritis by a famous rheumatologist, but I found his drugs too strong and did not feel better. So I showed it to another rheumatologist last month, who has reduced my arthritis drugs and has sent me to you to confirm his suspicion of a nerve problem instead."

As I spoke to him, I felt he was an anxious and possibly bordering on depression. Often his wife would supply the answer to a question posed to him or remind him of the right answer. He was even vague about the timing of his symptoms. He had initially told my assistant that he was suffering for the last two years, but when I asked, he casually said two to three years. That got me to asking him my favourite question. "When were you completely alright Mr Saraf? No symptoms at all."

Now he said, "I have been having acidity for many years". On probing deeper, the three of us realized that he had been unwell for many years and his symptoms went further and further behind in the past. He grudgingly accepted that he had been having difficulty falling asleep for many years. Then I used my strategy of asking specifically when it started. Before marriage? Soon after marriage, or much later? He was humming and hawing, when his wife said, "Didn't it start soon after we shifted residence?"

I latched onto this point and asked him the details, as I guessed this was significant. Then he told me that he used to live in a huge bungalow in a joint family and, 25 years ago, he and his family shifted out from this bungalow while his brother continued to live there!

I asked him, did the acidity also start then? He said, "No. That I have been having for years." With our mapping tool, we came to the conclusion that the acidity started around one year after his marriage and so it went back to almost 50 years.

"What do you mean by acidity, Mr Saraf?" I asked and pointing to his sternum, promptly he said, "Heartburn." I continued, "Do you get headache with the acidity?" He replied, "Of course! Always, and it often gets relieved after a vomit." On probing further, we got the following information. He used to get frequent headaches for many years, but for the last 10 years, he had daily headaches and used to take two painkiller tablets every day. Only last month, at the behest of his physician, did he reduce them to twice a week!

I proceeded to examine him and, as I had expected, I found no evidence of any arthritis or neuropathy. Over the last couple of years, he had got numerous blood tests done, all of which were borderline or normal. But since the clinical impression was arthritis, the borderline tests were used to support the diagnosis. The mind of the doctor had been made up and the tests were used to support his diagnosis; it did not matter they were really very very doubtful. He also had multiple MRIs, including the brain and spine, which were also normal.

Thus, I had a fairly educated person who was sent to me with a suspicion of a nerve disorder. But he had been labelled as having, and had received therapy for, arthritis for the last one year; he had not been sleeping well for the last 25 years, had frequent headaches for almost 50 years, and was getting daily headache for the last 10 years! Clinically, he had no evidence of arthritis, only subjective pain in his joints. But the long-standing pain in the head was ignored by the rheumatologist.

All his tests were normal and yet, now we were trying to fish for a nerve disorder! Unfortunately, he had not yet even been asked to see a psychologist or psychiatrist. Nobody had ever thought of the mind playing a role in his illness. It was quite obvious to me that his symptoms were due to depression probably triggered by his having to leave the house. Also, he was having migraine quite frequently for the last 50 years and it had turned into a chronic, daily headache in the last 10 years.

I asked him to do a nerve conduction test just to convince him and his referring rheumatologist that there would be no nerve problem. I also asked him to fill out a screening form for anxiety and depression. Although his nerve conduction tests were normal, his score on the anxiety and depression scale was extremely high. We discussed the results and I allowed him to take some time to understand how his mind was playing a crucial role in his bodily complaints. I recommended a psychologist and he was finally on the way to finding his answers.

Orthopaedics have another angle altogether when children get involved. Pediatric orthopaedics throws open a whole new set of challenges as the doctor has to deal with not only the child's emotional well-being but also that of the parents. In fact, many emotional disturbances are seen 'by proxy'. This is when, for example, a mother's stress and illness anxiety is transferred onto a child, and she cannot stop feeling that the child is in distress and needs medical attention right away. Here are a few cases from Dr Patwardhan, a leading pediatric orthopaedic surgeon.

## Case 2

It was a regular rushed morning at the Pediatric Orthopedic OPD when a young girl walked in with her mother. The child looked to be around eight, and both mother and daughter walked in without the usual haste of two people who had waited a long time for their turn to be seen. The child, in fact, seemed to walk cautiously, as if expecting pain any minute now.

As their history was revealed, I learnt that the child was indeed eight years old and the duo had come to me for a second (or fifth, as I would later learn), opinion for the child's 'flat foot'. If you are wondering about my use of quotation marks around the word 'flat foot', let me explain. A flat foot is usually not a disease. It is a variation in a person's physiology, just like blue or black eyes, golden or black hair, etc. It usually does not need intervention and cannot be corrected, no matter how hard a patient tries (unless surgical intervention is sought).

Coming back to the OPD room. It was warm indeed, but the child was sweating profusely. She seemed scared, more than in any pain. The mother started the dialogue:

Mother: Doctor, this is S., my only child. She has had severe pain in her legs for many months now. We have done everything possible to help her, but nothing seems to be working. The poor child was born with a flat foot and now the pain is constantly present.

Doc: Your file here mentions that you have tried orthotics in the past. Tell me more about them. How much did they help?

Mother: Oh, I don't think that doctor gave us the right footwear. We spent so much money on those insoles and wedges. Her pain only seems to be increasing.

Doctor: How many hours have you had her wear those shoes on a daily basis?

Mother: Doctor, I have tried my best to make her wear them. She wears them for only 10–15 minutes and then removes them. How will she ever improve?

Doc: So are the shoes faulty or the wearing time insufficient?

Mother: I assumed that such expensive shoes should have shown results earlier, isn't it? The ones I wore as a child cost nothing compared to these. And yet, I wore them just as my mother instructed.

Doc: Oh! So you have a flat foot as well?

Mother: Yes.

Doc: How long did you wear your 'special shoes?'

Mother: Well, almost 12 years! (Did I sense a fleeting sense of pride? Or wait, was that disappointment?)

Doc: How's your foot now?

Mother: Nothing changed doctor. It's still the same.

I asked the child to hop on to the examining table. Her neuro workup was okay. Flexibility was okay. She did have hyper-flexibility syndrome, which is a common cause for the arch to collapse when a person stands up.

Mother (While the child is being examined): She wakes up at night doctor. Crying. Says her legs are paining. I press her legs and she feels better. I read 'somewhere' that flat foot can cause this kind of pain.

Doctor (Now speaking directly to the child): Tell me, when does it hurt the most?

Child: When Mumma makes me wear those pokey shoes.

Doc: And other times?

Child: Sometimes at night.

Doc: During the day, how long do you wear the shoes?

Child: Mumma forces me to wear for a long time. But I can't bear the pain. So I keep removing them.

Doc: Come on then. Let's get you off the table.

I sat in front of a genuinely distraught mother, whose child was absolutely normal. Yes, there was nothing wrong with that eight-year-old child, at least physically. Her prolapsed arch was not causing any pain, but the orthotics were. The anxiety of not listening to her mother was also intense. The child was experiencing 'growing pains' which are common at her age. It had nothing to do with the flat foot.

Doc: After wearing your orthotics for 12 years, aren't you convinced by now that they don't work? Just let her be free. Throw away those shoes. Just an arch support in the shoes cannot create a permanent arch for her. This is a genetic predisposition that she has. There's nothing you should do about it. And her growing pains will pass too. It's normal for children at this age to experience such pains at night. They have nothing to do with the flat foot.

Mother: But doctor…isn't there any way to cure it? It's… umm…a bad omen for a girl in our community to have a flat foot. I don't want this to hamper her future.

Doc: Superstition has no medical cure. She needs no intervention, no treatment. She needs acceptance and the freedom to play in whatever shoes she chooses.

The mother looked upset and relieved in equal parts. The child was trying in vain to hide her glee. They left without a prescription, but with hope (hopefully!).

Flat foot is a phenomenon that is grossly misunderstood and over treated. Dr Benjamin Joseph from Manipal conducted a research and found that unshod feet have a better arch than people with shoes. Walking bare feet helps in strengthening the arch. Which is something most parents don't allow their children to do nowadays. Children wear shoes even before they learn to walk. No wonder the rates of collapsed arches are on the rise.

We treat flat foot only in some cases. If the child is a teen when the foot is fully grown, if it is unilateral, progressive, or is generally painful. Orthotics can be used to relieve the pain in such cases as they distribute the weight more evenly. An arch is not really created. Extreme cases call for surgical correction. The incidence of pathological flat foot is, in fact, only about 10%.

Medically speaking, the child had no disease. But was the pain real? Absolutely. The pain was as real as it would be after an injury. The anxiety that the child constantly felt with regards to the corrective footwear was two-fold. The first was the fear of the mother who insisted on wearing the uncomfortable shoes. The second was the preemptive pain i.e., hating the shoes because they would cause pain. This surety of pain helped the pain come on more swiftly. And this would create a constant state of turmoil in the child's mind. Understanding that the shoes were not a cure for the perceived deformity helped in effective pain management. And, as for the growing pains, well they just need to be outgrown.

Having spoken about this angle of psychosomatic pain, there is another case that comes to my mind immediately.

## Case 3

A morose 13-year-old boy was brought to the OPD by his parents. They looked tired, although it was still early in the day. He looked uninterested, almost dejected. The parents took the chairs and he sat on the leftover chair to the side, the patient's seat. It looked like they had done this many times before. It was almost like a rehearsed routine. As soon as I asked them what the problem was, he asked if he should get on to the examination table. I asked him to wait a bit till I oriented myself with his problem a little more.

The mother began, although I half expected the father to join in chorus. She crisply described his pain. The child had a pain in the left foot since 'forever'. He would wake up crying out with pain at night, sometimes, and she would give him an NSAID. The pain would subside and he would fall back asleep. Multiple opinions had revealed various probable causes. Flat foot, being the first. The second of a vitamin D deficiency which was promptly corrected. The pain continued. Orthotics gave no relief.

Doc: When does this pain bother him the most?

Father (Speaking almost instantly): Oh, it's usually during exams and tests. You know how stressful class eight can be. I think he isn't able to cope with the pressure.

Doc: Wow! You seem to be sure that this pain is caused by stress. Has anyone told you so?

Father: The last doctor said it was nothing. So it must be stress, na?

Doc: Let me see.

After examining the patient, I felt there was something purely organic about this pain. This was not psychosomatic at all. The child probably had an Osteoid

Osteoma. This hunch was later confirmed on a nuclear scan. An obvious diagnosis had been missed and the child had gone through the trauma of pain and blame.

The family came back the next day with the nuclear scan, which confirmed the diagnosis. We discussed radio frequency ablation as the first choice of treatment for the same. While we were discussing the treatment details, I noticed the teenager wipe a tear. He had found a reason for his pain. And he had been validated. He had been stressed, yes. But, in this case, the stress came after the disease. The pain and undiagnosed condition had left him feeling vulnerable and distraught. And when his parents saw him stressed, they promptly blamed the stress for his pain. A vicious circle entrapped them. Although his parents had started to believe that this was stress-induced pain, they didn't stop from seeking an expert opinion just to err on the side of caution. This is what made all the difference. The child was able to finally get a diagnosis. This is the perfect example of inclusivity. They did not exclude the possibility of an organic ailment even though they were rather sure it was purely psychosomatic. They left the final diagnosis and decision in the hands of a doctor they could trust, thus paving the way for healing. The treatment was simple, uneventful, and the child is now pain-free.

## Case 4

The next case is narrated by Dr Kinjal Goyal, from the commencement of psychotherapy till a substantial relief from symptoms is achieved.

"Ms L came to me, referred by her physician. She presented with intermittent severe pain in her shoulder, running down to her hand. When this pain would hit, it would make it impossible for her to continue doing what she had been doing at the time. She described the pain as sharp electrical jabs and also reported a 'dead' feeling in her hand, a sort of temporary paralysis. She was a bright student pursuing her medical degree and always scored top marks in her class. She was diligent and hardworking. She had visited neurologists (more than once), orthopaedics, general physicians, and had undergone a whole battery of tests, which, to her chagrin always turned out normal. Without even a trace of a diagnosis, no treatment was recommended. She was asked to continue her ongoing yoga classes and to maintain optimum hydration. Beyond this, there was nothing that was advised. When she had another debilitating 'episode' during her internal assessment papers, she decided to quit the exam and seek help once more. This time, her GP asked to seek psychotherapy.

Ms L came across as a rather calm person. She was courteous and had been punctual for her appointment. She described her symptoms with impressive detail and kept saying how badly the episodes were affecting her academically. She had done badly in her previous exams and although the teachers had been very supportive, she knew she would have to up her scores immediately if she were to do well in the finals and beyond. She was aware that she was a bright student and that a lot was riding on her academic performance.

After a few sessions, it was established that her episodes had a rough overlap with exams. As the sessions progressed, she learnt that her stress was not 'bad marks' but, in fact, 'flawless marks'. She couldn't stand the idea of not getting a perfect score. It would mean she was slipping up and letting her teachers and parents down. As the curriculum got more demanding, she started fearing a bad score. She wanted to do well. But the stress overwhelmed her. Through biofeedback, she learnt how the stress would affect her posture and how she would unknowingly clench various parts of her hand, including her shoulder, neck, and forearm. All this snowballed into excruciating pain, cramps, and the feeling of being paralysed. She was not making it up. The pain was real. The cramps were real. As she learnt various relaxation techniques, she started reporting a clear reduction in the pain. Through CBT, her fear and anxiety were dealt with and she felt confident once more, to sit for her exams. Through systematic desensitization, she felt less anxious thinking of the exams and calmer when faced with challenging questions. Slowly, she overcame the whole ordeal and is now symptom-free."

## Conclusion

Orthopaedics is thus a complicated playing field for psychosomatic pain. Whilst it is easier for most to accept an accelerated heart rate due to stress, or even a heavy head due to prolonged anxiety, it is very hard for doctors and patients alike to believe that emotional disturbances can cause such 'obviously' physical pain. It is, therefore, most effective to use the biopsychosocial model when treating orthopaedic-psychosomatic manifestations. Further research into the field will hopefully pave the way for more understanding and a wider acceptance.

# CHAPTER 11
# Oncology: A Matter of Growth

~With Dr Bhooshan Ranade
and Dr Manish Agarwal

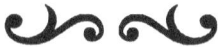

The very word cancer evokes fear and insecurity, some of it justified, some not. Cancer is not one disease but a group of over 100 diseases, in which some of the body cells start to divide and grow excessively and uncontrollably, spreading into the surrounding as well as distant areas.

There are different types of cancer, depending on which organ or which tissue it arises from; for example, lung cancer when it arises in the lung or leukemia when it arises in the blood forming tissue or bone marrow.

Many cancers are preventable and many are treatable, particularly in the early stages. Cancer happens due to a combination of genetic predispositions as well as exposure to various cancer inducing agents like radiation or smoking. In some situations, the exact cause of the cancer may never be found.

To estimate the prognosis and plan the treatment, doctors consider the grade and the stage of the cancer as well as the age and the general condition of the patient. The grade of the cancer is a measure of how bad the cancer looks under the microscope; the more abnormal it looks the more likely is it to be aggressive and spread and less likely to respond to therapy. The stages measure the spread; varying from no spread to severe spread.

## The mind and cancer

Let us now look at the interaction of the mind with cancer. Cancer is seen by many as an enemy. People often speak of it as a person, out to kill you silently and inexorably. Lay press and movies also reinforce this view of cancer being silent, difficult to treat or even untreatable. A person facing cancer is said to be fighting it, as if it is a battle to be won.

Yes, certain personality styles can lead to risky behavior like smoking. Similarly, a tenacious attitude may help you in accepting all that goes with cancer therapy. But there is no real evidence that a personality trait or inadequate coping style, stress by itself or by affecting your immunity, or depression or grief, can cause cancer or make you more likely to die from it. It is worth having a positive attitude when one does get diagnosed with cancer but that does not mean that you cannot feel afraid, angry or depressed. These are natural feelings and one cannot be made to feel guilty for getting these thoughts or feelings. It is unrealistic to expect a person to remain positive always and throughout. In fact, a crucial part of managing cancer is to enquire about and pay attention to the emotional state of the patient at every stage.

There are endless cases of people with sunny dispositions and extremely positive attitudes succumbing to cancer. A positive attitude can help deal with the disease but in no way can it be thought to be a complete prevention or cure.

Social support is crucial for a good outcome in the treatment of most diseases. Cancer is no different. There are, however, many layers of secrecy around a diagnosis of cancer which can make it hard for a patient and his/her family to seek help and receive the required support. It is not uncommon for a family to ask to speak to the doctor alone, asking the patient to step out, so that the patient can be kept 'safe' from the distressing diagnosis. Many people assume that the patient will suffer emotionally and probably simply break down if they are told that they have cancer. They attempt to protect their loved one by hiding the diagnosis. However, this stops the patient from being able to talk about their fears. Eventually, the patient finds out what the true nature of the disease is. However, as no one talks about it in front of them or with them, they need to face the fears and treatment alone, without having anyone to confide in. In some cases, the family refuses to share a cancer diagnosis with friends and extended family. This works well for some, offering privacy and a time to heal, but again, does not allow the suffering family to lean on others for the much-needed emotional support.

Dr Ranade:

As an oncologist, I see fear before the patient comes face to face with real pain. I can think of various other ailments where the prognosis is grimmer than initial stage cancers; but in no other disease does the diagnosis itself elicit as much fear and distress as in cancer. It is complicated to try and justify the reputation that cancer has earned. Some of my patients come back and tell me that they can't decide what was worse, the disease or the treatment. Some, however, do very well with treatment, be it surgery, chemotherapy or a combination of various treatment modalities. Some patients tide over the cancer and resume life as before, while some survive but only as mere shadows of their previous selves. Sometimes, lives are lost. Cancer treatment can take a toll not only on the patient, but on the caregivers as well. Promises of a cure abound outside the field of medicine. One of the main fallacies that people fall prey to, is the over generalization of all cancers as the same disease. Hence, if one person had, say a benign or grade 1 tumour, he or she would have recovered very well with allopathic treatment. If however, this patient tries out an alternative therapy and heals, everyone in his or her close and not so close circle will believe that all cancers can be cured by the said alternative treatment. This is where things start to go wrong. If, now, someone who has a stage 3 or 4 malignant tumour and needs surgery and chemotherapy urgently, he may be more inclined towards the alternative treatment plan that worked so well for his friend mentioned above. This can not only endanger his life, but also make it harder to trust the doctor who is recommending the 'unpleasant and painful' treatment options. Apart from trust, there are a multitude of factors that come into play where cancer treatment is involved. A patient's body undergoes a physically visible transformation and can be the object of discussion even among well-meaning friends and family. The fear of the unknown reigns supreme. Also, the patient feels a sense of helplessness as an unwanted mass grows at will inside the body that he thought he had full control over.

A few cases come to my mind as soon as I think about the power of the human mind in the healing process.

## Case 1

It was an unusually hot May in 2004. But well, I probably say that for every summer I see in Pune. Mr H walked in with a young girl, probably close to him in age and both had beads of perspiration on their foreheads. I made a quick mental note to check on the air conditioning in the waiting room later that evening. Mr H introduced himself in crisp, impeccable English and also added with a happy smile that this was his wife of three months, Mrs J. She looked young and scared. She was clasping a folder probably containing the reports that Mr H had come to discuss with me.

It was very hard to believe that this charming young man had just received a diagnosis of advanced colonic cancer and was here to discuss his treatment options. I told myself that he probably didn't understand the risks and bleak prognosis, but I was taken aback once again, when he candidly discussed all the known (and some rare) risks of his disease and treatment. I felt my face mirroring the expression on Mrs J's face. I was worried about this young man. Surgery was the first step, but I wasn't sure how far it would take him on the path of a cure. I told him as much and he seemed to take a minute to fully comprehend what I was saying. "Do you mean, doctor, that surgery may not work?" I tried to sound more confident than I felt, but honesty got the better of me. "We can't be 100% sure of how far the cancer has spread. Surgery will help us explore the colon and assess the tumour. If we are lucky, we will excise the tumour right then".

What he said next, made me see him in a whole new light. He looked his wife in the eye and said, "Did you hear that? The doctor is on my team now! He didn't say If I get lucky.. he said if we get lucky... I couldn't have asked for more at this point, really." His enthusiasm wasn't in the least infectious and she maintained her stoic state of extreme anxiety. My heart reached out to her. And to him.

The surgery was planned for the day after the next. It didn't take the surgeon too long to realise that the tumour was too large and the cancer too widespread to allow an excision. This tumour was inoperable. They shifted him out to recovery. I saw him that evening, dragging my feet and lowering my eyes. His wife seemed sadder, shrunken, as if she had a terrible ailment, and deathly quiet. He was in pain from the surgery, but his demeanor was still as vibrant as a recovery room in a hospital might permit.

Mr H: Thank you for suggesting the surgery right away doctor. At least we know that it's not our best option now.

Doc: I am sorry, H. I truly am. I was hoping the tumour would be more contained. Unfortunately, it was not the case. The surgeons tried their best, but eventually had to take a call to leave the tumour untouched.

Mr H: What does that mean for me now doc? How do we move ahead? The surgeon was nice enough to answer me when I asked him what he thought of my 'time left on earth'. But honestly, I think he's wrong. Three months, he said. I don't want to count the days to my death, half-heartedly ticking off my bucket list. I want to fight this cancer. I know I can.

Doctor: I respect your will to do so H. You are young and fit otherwise. Would you like a second opinion on this?

Mr H: I don't mind if you wish to discuss possibilities with others in your field doc. I don't need a second opinion for myself. I know I am with the right doctor.

Doc: Alright then. Let's do this. You need some time to allow the incisions to heal. Until then, I shall come up with the best way forward. I am sure you are aware that it won't be easy. In fact, it will be really hard. But I am sure there is something we can try. And H, I cannot promise anything. Except that I will try my best.

Mr H: That's pretty much all that I need doc.

He gave me a weak smile as I left his room. I nodded in Mrs J's direction, but she was too disturbed to respond.

We formulated a treatment plan of intensive chemotherapy and radiation. Mr H started his treatment and braved the chemicals coursing through his body. His smile was strong sometimes, weak sometimes, but it always lingered. His next set of scans showed that the chemotherapy had helped to shrink the tumour to a size that was now operable. His surgery went off well and the surgeon was able to excise the entire tumour this time. He followed up with more chemo and radiation and to our utter amazement, his cancer vanished from the scans. We stayed on the side of caution and repeated his scans at regular intervals to ensure that the cancer did not return as a nasty shock. It stayed away.

Another unusually hot summer day, in May 2018, H walked in with his wife, carrying a gift box for me. It contained sweets that his mother had sent, for she celebrated his return from inevitable death each May. A man who had been given three months to live, continues to be healthy and disease free, 15 years after. His smile is the same. His wife's smile is brighter though. His enthusiasm did end up rubbing off on all of us finally!

In the case discussed above, the patient was given a grave diagnosis and told that he probably didn't have a very long time left to live. Although, at first, it seems like his positive attitude and grit helped him overcome this terrible disease, there's more to it than just an attitude. The trust he had in his doctor helped him stay away from pseudo therapies. His will to overcome allowed him to choose different treatment options with his doctor's advice as time passed by, thereby increasing his chances of survival and healing. His emotional state by itself didn't cure him of the cancer. It did, however, act as a catalyst in creating a suitable environment for his treatment.

Dr Manish Agarwal:

## Case 2

Mr M, a 59 year old man was referred to me in 2009 august with a painful forearm swelling. He looked like a very intelligent and fit man. His brother-in-law was a colleague and had told me that he was a very high IQ person who has been an international bridge champion. I saw his x-rays and his MRI and thought that this was a malignant tumor arising from the radius, one of his forearm bones. He gave a strong history of smoking and I was worried that this could be lung cancer which had spread to the bone. His chest x-ray was clear so we did a needle biopsy on him. The biopsy confirmed that this was a metastatic carcinoma probably from the lung. We confirmed this with a PET-CT scan which showed a small mass in his lung which was the source of this larger forearm tumor. There was no disease anywhere else. We sat down in my office for counseling and I revealed to him that he had stage 4 lung cancer which has an average survival of six months or less. To my surprise, he was unfazed, well prepared to face this news. He asked what was the way ahead. We had two options: to fight the disease with an attempt to cure with a very low chance of success (<5% chance at that time) or accept the defeat and aim to do only what was necessary to relieve his pain and give him a quality of life. Mr M was intelligent enough to be able to make his own decision. He decided to fight, which meant chemotherapy followed by two major surgeries to remove completely the lung and forearm tumors. All this knowing that the odds of winning were <5%. He did not once look depressed, he never asked "why me?". I immediately realized that I was treating an exceptionally positive man. His forearm surgery required to think out of the box as apart from being a bridge player, he was a carrom champion (I'm told that you rarely got the striker back to play once he had a chance, he would clear the board). We planned to remove his tumor affected bone and replace it with a special custom-made titanium implant so that I could save his joint part and still have a strong grip on the bone. This implant was ordered from London, would take six weeks to be made so we started him on chemotherapy. Post chemotherapy scans showed a very good response. We did his forearm surgery and lung surgery. I was certain that with his mental strength, he would recover well which he did. Today he is a long term survivor with no sign of disease. He is fully functional, works long hours as a journalist and a writer. He was able to beat the odds with his attitude.

*In this case, again, the patient's attitude helped the doctor chart out a treatment plan which was out of the box. His chances for survival were slim without such dramatic intervention and it was his trust and willingness to go to the end of the road to get the best treatment possible that gave him a better shot at survival.*

## Case 3

Miss Z, was a pretty 21 year old girl from Guwahati, who came to me with pain and swelling around her left knee. She seemed anxious and hopeful at the same time. The anxiety stemmed from the fact that her primary doctor had suspected a bone cancer. She was accompanied by her brother, who seemed just as scared. I reviewed her X-rays and MRI and agreed with her primary doctor. We did a biopsy which confirmed an *Osteosarcoma* (bone cancer).

We did a PET scan which showed that the bone was the only site. This diagnosis was revealed to her. We told her that she would need chemotherapy and then surgery. She would lose all her hair with chemotherapy and surgery would involve removing 40% of her thigh bone with the knee joint and replacing it with a metallic implant.

She was devastated and cried for a long time. Once she had regained her composure a little, she asked me a single question: "Will I ever walk 'normally and will my hair grow back?" I confessed that she had a 60% chance of being cured, her hair would grow back but may not be the same as now and she would walk well if she did her physiotherapy. She would not be allowed to run or jump and that the metallic joint would not last forever and would need replacement in future.

Very unwillingly, she got admitted for chemotherapy. I had a feeling that she would be calling on me quite frequently during her hospital stay. And I was right. Her anxiety did warrant the attention and I knew she was battling more demons in the form of fear and anxiety than just the chemicals in the chemo. She asked me each time she met me if she would walk normally again. Every time I reassured her knowing in my mind that she may have a limp. She went through surgery and then started walking with the aid of a walker. As time passed, she grew stronger and more confident. She started walking well. She wanted so badly to have a normal gait, it became her superpower. She spent more time and effort in physiotherapy to ensure that she doesn't have a limp.

A year after her chemotherapy completion, she sent me several photographs from her modeling session. I was pleasantly surprised. She had regained her confidence, was looking beautiful and more importantly was confident. She then confided to me that she wanted to be an airhostess. I was concerned. Would her scar and weak leg from surgery be a handicap? I told her to go ahead and apply. I got a worried call a few months later. She was in tears. She said that in the next few days, she would have to undergo a fitness test where she was required to jump onto the aeroplane slide and then get up quickly after she was on ground. I told her not to worry, she would be able to do it. I wasn't sure she would clear it. But I wasn't even sure she wouldn't. I stayed on the side of optimism and told her to go for it. She cleared the test and sent me the video. Today she flies both domestic and international sectors on one of the top airlines and no one can tell that she has gone through so much treatment for cancer. She lives alone and also supports her family (she was from a low middle-class family which I am sure was in debt after her treatment). Her strong desire to become an airhostess made her recover well. Her desire to walk normally, to have normal hair and to not look like a cancer patient took her a long way in achieving her goals.

**We were able to speak to the patient whose case this was. As a psychologist, I was interested in knowing the other side of the story too. Here are some excerpts from what the patient wrote in:**

*The mind plays a very important role in healing. I used to tell myself every day that I am getting better, to make my body believe it. For me, the diagnosis was the hardest moment; I believed, as most people do, that with cancer, death is certain. Having a doctor who understood my fears and supported me during the toughest time was as important as the treatment itself. I rely heavily on my family for support but I realized that at times like this, family members are scared and heartbroken themselves. They also rely on the doctor. My surgeon never once showed annoyance at my endless questions and answered me patiently each time I called upon him.*

*I had good days and bad days too. On the days I was low, I would allow myself to cry and then collect my energies and focus only on healing.*

Everyday, I see lots of people, young and old diagnosed and treated for cancer. I am very sure that the outcomes are greatly affected by the mind. A strong desire to win, an ability to stay calm and focused, clearly improves outcomes. I don't have hard numbers, but I do feel that negative and depressed people end up with more complications and worse outcomes. Children have much better outcome than adults, I believe this is more from a mental attitude rather than physical differences. A child is focused on only one thing: when can they go back to play with their friends. They trust their parents, they are not bothered about chance of death. Miss Z, who was very childlike in her attitude could do well because of it. Mr M was a strong mind capable of avoiding the stress and emotional overlay and could take his own decisions. We now know scientifically that mind controls our immune system which fights all disease including cancer. Time to make psychotherapy a part of our treatment. Although as a doctor and a human being, it is heart breaking to see so many beautiful lives lost to cancer, it is also heartwarming and encouraging to encounter some people who harness the power of the mind to give themselves the best chance of beating the disease. This is, of course, not to say that those who didn't make it had a negative attitude. Unfortunately, sometimes, the strongest mind and the best attitude may also fall short. Cancer is complicated. The emotions attached with it are complex. Not only during the diagnosis phase, but also during the treatment and post treatment phase, do emotions run high. Trust, grit and optimism are known to improve outcomes, but sometimes, aggressive forms of the disease beat them too. There is still a lot to learn and discover in the field of psycho-oncology and hopefully, in the future, we will be better able to harness the power of the mind in dealing with cancers.

One of the hardest things that patients find in receiving a cancer diagnosis is accepting that the fateful disease happened to them. Psychotherapeutic intervention helps in various stages. First, acceptance and compliance with the suggested treatment plan. Second, battling depression and anxiety during the course of the treatment, which may be painful and take over the patient's life completely for a while. A patient's body image also changes as the medicines and disease together change the reflection a patient sees in the mirror. Third, even if a patient is able to beat the disease and has been given the all-clear from doctors, some might suffer from Post Traumatic Stress Disorder while some may live in the constant fear of the disease recurring. Therapy helps tremendously in this stage, helping a patient battle anxiety and regain confidence and self efficacy.

Caregivers also need emotional support. Sometimes, seeing a close friend or family member suffer from and succumb to cancer can spark sudden illness anxiety. It can be exhausting providing end of life care to someone and taking care of oneself takes a back seat. Helping caregivers cope is as important as helping the patient. Again, various forms of psychotherapy are used effectively to help overcome this phase.

Cancer is a dreaded disease. At an advanced stage, or if it an aggressive cancer, it can be fatal, with the patient suffering through immense pain during treatment. New research is improving outcomes in a few areas, but a lot is yet to be done to take the fear away from the dreaded disease. Our language around cancer has gradually evolved to show respect and honour those who have healed from cancer. We call them survivors, those who have won the battle. Those who fought valiantly. The truth is, the ones who didn't make it to the other end of the tunnel were no less valiant. They did not abandon the battle. They simply had cancers which took over their bodies faster than medicines could push back.

Taking care of a patient's mental wellbeing may help with the healing process. It may also help them by giving them space to heal emotionally while the body tries to overcome the cancer. Emotional strength may not completely prevent cancer or offer a full recovery when diagnosed with it, but it can make a difference to the outcome in some cases. The mind is, in that sense, a very important aspect for the treatment of cancer.

# Conclusion

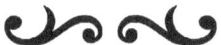

When we started this book, it was the year 2018. The world had not seen a pandemic in living memory and mental health issues were still fairly taboo. As we neared the end of our writing, the year was 2020. As this book goes into print, the world is battling the Covid19 Pandemic and nothing seems the same anymore. New 'normals' are being established. Mental health is being spoken about. There has been a sudden rise in cases of Illness Anxiety Disorder, amongst other mental health disorders. Yet, at the heart of it, our book remains what we intended it to be: an amalgamation of thoughts, feelings and experiences of leading doctors in various fields, with regards to psychosomatics.

Blind to the Mind can be best defined by listing what it is not. It is not an attempt to distinguish the mind from the body. It is not an attempt to classify 'real' vs 'not so real' diseases. It is not about mind-body dualism at all. In fact, it is just the opposite. This book is an attempt to see the mind and body as a whole and to understand how the mind plays a vital role in the disease-illness axis across various ailments.

As you have now realised, this is not a medical textbook. We do not claim to have the cure for any ailment blindly through psychotherapy. We do not wish to undermine the clinical opinion of a doctor and urge our readers to use this book as a tool for opening their minds, not as a way of second guessing their doctors. We also hope that all the doctors who read this book will be able to start the conversation about psychosomatics with their peers and patients more seamlessly.

Although we have tried to cover as many fields as we could, we obviously cannot claim to have covered them all. That would have been logistically impossible and would have still left us with some fields we never thought of. Gynecology, nephrology, general medicine, dermatology etc. are some of the large fields that are conspicuous by their absence here. Hopefully, we shall cover them soon, on some other platform.

We hope that whether you are a medical professional, a patient or someone who is simply keen on finding out how our mind can hamper or foster healing, between the covers of 'Blind to the Mind', you have found the answers that you have been seeking.

www.ingramcontent.com/pod-product-compliance
Lightning Source LLC
Chambersburg PA
CBHW020905180526
45163CB00007B/2626